Advance Praise

"Deanna shines a light on what would otherwise be kept hidden in the dark. It is extremely eye-opening the number of cases she shares as just ONE practitioner. I would recommend this book for any health care worker who is in direct patient care."

~ Holly Peterson, RN

"Direct from the front lines of clinical Care, an experienced nurse Practitioner chronicles significant adverse events from COVID jabs she observed in her patients. The ability of clinicians to detect changes in patterns of illness and clinical deterioration temporally associated with COVID jabs should serve as early warning signs of troubling problems with novel COVID injections."

~ Elizabeth Mumper, MD, FAAP, IFMCP, President and CEO, Advocates for Children and the Rimland Center for Integrative Medicine

GASOLINE

Observations after New COVID
Inoculations, in Layman's Terms

DEANNA L. KLINE, AGNP-C, MSN, RN

Contents

Copyrighted Materials

Dedication

This book is dedicated to every person worldwide who has experienced new, often sudden, or worsened serious health issues due to the introduction of spike protein via inoculations. It is also dedicated to many people I care about, and attempted to warn. Spike protein is a protein on the surface of the SARS-Cov-2 virus, which builds up in the body during a COVID illness, and which is produced in the body from the effects of COVID inoculations.

If you are suffering, or worse, lost a loved one, I'm so very sorry. Please believe me, I grieve with you.

Historically trusted yet thickly veiled organizations, community pillars, and even the most prestigious medical research journals and health care organizations are conflicted and are the subject of much controversy. Many **are** shouting an alert, but powerful enigmas create and steer what is heard. The powerful who rule media cancel and ridicule thousands of scientists and medical doctors as well as those who share their experiences despite **not** having the illness. Millions of people around the world have suffered, and this book is a **tiny sampling** of them. Let us never forget those who did not survive.

Many thanks to the doctors, nurses, scientists, lawyers, and people from all walks of life who reassured me I wasn't alone.

Thank you, also, to Kathryn Mills and Gail McClemore.

The most abundant thanks go to those who asked to include their stories here.

Introduction

This book is filled with real people who suffered or died shortly after receiving the new COVID inoculations. This book is **not** a complete scientific theory or literature review, though it references current research. The accounts shared in this book are from clinical observations in primary care practice from **February 2021 to February 2022 only**. *Please keep that in mind when you are reading. It was difficult to stop writing, as I continue to see people in similar situations since their booster, in 2022.*

I had every scheduled childhood vaccine, received many vaccines while serving in the Air Force, and got dozens of flu shots over the years. I encourage you to get all the shots you desire, research until you are satisfied, and read outside of your AI trained feed and favorite channel. The decision to use a medication or get a vaccine or try experimental therapies is yours alone. This book is about observations after COVID inoculations, because they are new, were trialed for a very short time, and because I saw many trends of ill effects. I did not think the government, large healthcare corporations, or medical schools were going to study these effects, or if they did, that results wouldn't be widely or completely shared. I also read one clinical trial from one company that received the emergency use authorization (EUA) for their product, and found many more adverse effects than were discussed in it, day after day in my patients. It is *not* about being pro- or anti-vaccine. Realize there are millions of people, perhaps a billion or more worldwide, who prefer to choose their particular vaccine acceptance based on their own research and decisions, as well as their own personal, familial, and professional risks and benefits. Some choose none and some choose all. Some people choose a few vaccines and delay a few others to a certain age or until they enter a certain occupation.

Resist the urge to lump every single person in the world into pro- or anti-vaccine camps, as if there is only two, and opposing, options for vaccination and medication. Realize that when a person gets diagnosed with any number of diseases, there are different options for treatment and yes, even several different options for medication to address that same disease or symptom. The treatment, prevention, or medication may be different among dozens of people. We have hundreds of options for herbal tea, caffeine, clothing, hair color, jewelry, tattoos, exercise or lack thereof, hobbies, sports, vehicles, leisure, entertainment, investments, athletic shoes, substance use and abuse, lotions, potions, oils, vitamins, supplements, medicines, and chiropractors, massage therapists, functional medicine providers, spiritual gurus, priests, pastors, coaches, personal trainers, teachers, lawyers, naturopathic providers, conventional doctors, nurses, therapists, dietitians, holistic providers, physiatrists and psychiatric help. To each their own, friends. Truly, millions of us don't agree 100% on every single issue in the world with our spouse or sibling, but we still love each other and often make effort to understand one another.

Will this book contribute to potential new understanding, gained from these precious people and changes in their body and health? These new health concerns began in perilous proximity to the dates of their shots. Some readers and critics will say they just had covid antibodies, so these health problems were just covid complications and not shot complications. I will say no, this is not the case, because some were tested, and others I actually treated for covid illness months *after their* mRNA injection and *well after* their side effects occurred.

Some people will mock and dismiss the accounts represented by the real people in this book. However, I ask, are people's health complaints, lab results, CT results, new and unexpected diagnoses, corroborating collective symptoms, pain, and *skyrocketing medical visits* falsehoods? Are people *labeled liars because someone disagrees?* When someone disagrees, what *explanation* is offered? Can it negate the effects to these people's health and lives? Is *actual* debate taking place, or just canceling and mocking?

To address those questions, hundreds of studies are cited at the end of this book and are weighted on a scale of some proof and truths. *I invite you to read them.* To date, facts reveal *clots and myocarditis have a definite connection to the vaccine, as do inflammation, heart risks, and lymph node swelling.* Beyond these, we don't know; the science could take years. Truthfully, we may never know. For now, you'll have to search deeply, far and wide, beyond your evening news, social media, and the first pages of the most popular search engines. You might have to change browsers and consider news sources you've never heard of before. You'll likely have to venture out, far away from all you once trusted and believed. I had to, but I started doing it twenty-two years ago as an inquisitive nurse, so I had a jump start on 2020. It didn't make it easier to swallow, though. Still, you must decide if seeking the hard truths, where reconciliation and learning come, enlighten, and create change, are worth it to you, your loved ones, and humanity.

Did you notice that emergency rooms and urgent care clinics were packed all summer in 2021? They were packed all spring and summer of 2021, which is especially bizarre for that time of year. There was much less COVID illness and hospitalization in the spring and summer. What places were packed in late winter and spring 2021? Mass vaccination centers.

For years, I heard the nearby ambulance pull out about twice a week, occasionally three times a week. Similarly, I would see *one or fewer* ER or hospitalization follow-up patients per week, for years.

Beginning in the spring of 2021, the ambulance pulled out **three to six times every single day**. I also then began to see post hospitalization or post urgent care visit patients daily, and sometimes two a day, rather than once a week like prior years.

Chances are, you know someone who was hospitalized in 2021. Some of course, especially in winter, were admitted for COVID. *I'm so sorry if you lost someone you loved to this. I did as well.* I pray you have peace. Sadly, the people I know who passed were not offered any early treatment, even high risk people who desperately needed early treatment. I'm so sorry. It is such a tragedy. Believe me, *I grieve with you.*

Still, many others were *not* hospitalized for COVID in the spring, summer, and fall of 2021. Not all ER and hospital visits were COVID illnesses. Was everyone you know who went to the hospital in 2021 only admitted for COVID? I can confidently tell you the answer is **no**. How do I know they weren't all COVID? Because I often read emergency room encounter notes, hospital admission and discharge summaries, and see people afterward at their follow-up primary care visit. Many new trends emerged, and continue to land people in the hospital. Why haven't others who have read the same documents not sounded the alarm? A good question indeed, and one to ponder.

I have left many people I suspected had a reaction to the shots out of this book because other causes or contributing factors could not be as easily ruled out. The cases chosen for this book were selected under scrutiny. This book only covers the first 12 months since the new shots were introduced. There were more people I could have included, but it seems I would never stop writing the book if I kept adding people who suffered after later boosters. There are no patient identifiers mentioned anywhere in this book, and this book is not about workups or treatments for potential reactions, although I may mention a few. This book is about people whose lives have changed or were lost.

In 2021, I have often said, "spike protein is spike protein, I don't care how you get it" and it turns out there are some similar effects and mechanisms that can take place in some people, **no matter how spike protein is obtained** (1,2,3). A couple of months into mass inoculations, I added another phrase, "It's gasoline on your one flame of inflammation". This appears quite true for many and it is commonly known that SARS-Cov-2 creates a state of escalating inflammation as the illness progresses. I've had dozens of people whose baseline laboratory inflammatory related markers, the ESR (Erythromycin Sedimentation Rate) and/or hs-CRP (High Sensitivity C-Reactive Protein) are low normal or in the middle normal range for years, and then during or after the illness, **OR after the spike protein is produced** in their body from covid mRNA injections, they are elevated and in some cases very elevated. These markers do not diagnose anything specific, they simply reveal that a certain level of inflammation or health risks, are in the body. *The more these markers are elevated, potentially the more pain or the more inflammatory related illness and disease presents itself. This will look different in each person depending on the persons inflammatory status and problem locations of pain or inflammatory disease in the body, making them worse or newly show up.* Now, I add, "I'm sad for susceptible spines and brains" and "It's the trigger on your immune deficiency". Later in this book, you will see why.

The following chapters will reveal real people who did **not** have the illness but obtained the spike protein via the mechanism of the injection. Lovely, kind, fabulous people.

I have seen **one** person with a pulmonary embolus (blood clot in the lung) after COVID illness. I have also seen over a dozen with "brain fog", fatigue or lingering upper respiratory symptoms. I am also aware of several of the laboratory blood count, chemistry, enzyme, and inflammation changes that take place during the illness and as one recovers, because I have treated people in their covid illness, both vaccinated and unvaccinated. Recently, *we are told that new, long COVID symptoms may first present some time later in the months following covid illness* (4), perhaps explaining why a few people have new or worsened health problems after the illness. I believe the same is true for many people in the months following receiving these mRNA injections, as spike protein continues to affect the organs and vessels, which is different from all prior vaccines in our lifetimes. Booster shots then add to this, or potentially create an autoimmune response onto the area of the body infiltrated and altered by spike protein from the first two shots.

The people in this book had received mRNA, which produced spike protein in their body, but did **not** have a history of COVID or current COVID illness. Yet, significant complications occurred, in some cases, soon after injection and, in other cases, weeks to months afterward. For example, we now know that heart and circulation risks are doubled due to endothelial inflammation for *at least 10 weeks* after the injections (4). Endothelial tissue is the lining on the inside of your blood vessels. The study providing the information was stopped after 10 weeks, so we don't yet know how long the increased heart attack or vascular risk remains after injection. Even Pfizer's release of the post-marketing analysis revealed effects occurring eight weeks later (5), and again, more extended research periods have yet to be performed. We may not learn how many months post-inoculation adverse effects may occur for several years. I have an idea, because I continue to see these trends in the summer of 2022.

Further, why aren't all the new studies related to all things post COVID identifying who was vaccinated and who was not in them? I believe the narrative has already been set to say that all the recent health declines are from post-COVID illness alone. *This is impossible to determine when research, data collection, and the onset of disease and death do not disclose whether there was COVID illness, COVID shots, or both.* Some are paying attention to life insurance claims. It has been over 18 months since the first COVID shot was given in the US. Why haven't studies been released to the public on the morbidity and mortality of the vaccinated compared to the unvaccinated in these emerging patterns of illness and death trends? Have they even begun? Will the results be truthful? Good questions.

I am one provider. Approximately 300,000 primary care providers existed in the US in 2010 (6). Now extrapolate the people one provider has seen across the nation, then try to do so worldwide. I estimate I have seen about 250 people with adverse reactions, but I will be generous and not count them due to less certainty and some other possible contributors. Confidently, I can say I have seen 100 people. If there were approximately 100 people with adverse events in 2021 and 300,000 providers, that would equal *30,000,000* people in the US alone. And this is only routine primary care providers, not emergency rooms or urgent clinics. Is there any wonder why both long-term care disability claims are rising, and all-cause deaths in 18-64 are up 40% for 2021? (7,8). The UK reported the same facts (9). A large German insurance company has also sounded the alarm on massive rates of side effects (10). "Factcheckers" want to deny excess deaths or label excess deaths covid related and the same goes for life-changing side effects, even though the FDA itself listed most of the possible side effects, similar to what I discuss in this book, in their working list way back in ***October 2020*** (11).

Perhaps, like me, you know nurses or other medical professionals who gave their all and went to New York or other insanely busy cities to help in COVID hospitals. Perhaps, like me, you know medical doctors in some states have been warned by their state boards of medicine to not give medical exemptions for this new injection. I know others who work in different states and shared many challenging, painful, and tumultuous issues surrounding COVID care and treatment. I know several people who told me very recently that their doctor finally acknowledged the shots were the very likely cause of their numerous new health problems in the last year. The issues in this book are complicated, and we must face them no matter the horrific pain and stress each of us has faced in the last two years. If we don't, we are potentially feeding unnecessary **additional** injury and illness in millions of people, our peers and professions, and our families, friends, neighbors, and communities. If we don't, we possibly permit the crippling of children, generations, and nations. May we ever seek, study, learn, and be able to freely discuss and face the hard things in what is found today and in the future. May we discuss, debate, and study as adults rather than just repeat the sponsored evening news, insult, or hide.

This book is filled with real people. I encourage you to read about them.

Chapter 1

PEOPLE WITH CLOTS - STROKE (CLOT
OR BLEED IN THE BRAIN), TRANSIENT
ISCHEMIC ATTACK (TIA ANOTHER
NAME FOR MINI-STROKE),
THROMBOSIS (CLOT), PULMONARY
EMBOLUS (CLOT IN THE LUNG), AND
MICRO-CLOTS (MICROSCOPIC CLOTS,
OFTEN NOT SEEN ON IMAGING)

Middle Aged Woman – Stroke, Swollen Lymph Nodes

A thin, healthy, active woman in her early 50s took no medications
but had a history of migraine headaches as a young woman. She
complained of falling apart since her second shot. She stated she
began having many health problems a few days later. She volunteered this information. I did not specifically ask. She reported mild
right-sided face, arm, and leg numbness. She had a feeling of being
unsteady on her feet. She had a vague headache, nothing like her
typical migraines as a young lady. She now had recurrent sinus
infections. She saw an Ear, Nose, and Throat (ENT) doctor for the
sinus issues and discussed the face numbness and ongoing swollen
lymph nodes in her neck. The ENT told her to get another neurologist because her recent MRI revealed a cerebellar stroke, but the
neurologist continued to address only migraines. Cerebellar strokes
typically cause poor balance, being unsteady on one's feet. She
developed swollen lymph nodes in her groin many months later

while the neck nodes persisted. She was not asked the dates of her shots by neurology or urgent care visit providers.

You can read more about lymph nodes later in Chapter 16.

Elderly Woman – Transient Ischemic Attack (TIA) & First-degree Atrioventricular Block (AVB)

A mildly overweight woman in her 70s who did not smoke and took one medication and a few vitamins received her first shot at the end of March. Two days after her second shot, she went to the ER for what she called a spell and was released home. She never had any spells in the past. She had another spell of reduced mental awareness, confusion, and posterior head and neck pain with a fall two days later. She returned to the ER and was again released to go home. Possible diagnoses were a seizure, a Transient Ischemic Attack (TIA), a syncopal episode, or fainting of undetermined cause. Less than one week later, she was admitted to the hospital for a complete workup due to another potential TIA episode that lasted longer than the previous event. She was sent for lab, cardiac and neurological workups and imaging, including EEG, MRIs, and CT scans. Everything was negative, except her EKG. Her EKG showed a new first-degree atrioventricular block (AVB), but her heart remained in a normal rhythm.

A first-degree AVB is oftentimes not a problem, and people can live with it for years. Other times, people can experience symptoms when various heart blocks occur. She may have had it, or it may have been new; we don't know. TIAs do not create lasting stroke effects, such as a permanent weak leg, cognitive loss, or trouble swallowing, and they do not show up on CT scans or MRIs after the short-lived, transient events. She was not asked the dates of her shots in the ER. She still complains of unusual fatigue and brain fog. I suspect micro-clots or blood pressure escalations caused her to have the three TIAs.

You will see more about high- blood pressure in the next chapter.

Elderly Woman – Clots

An active and average-weight woman in her 70s who took no medications complained of a sudden onset of a lump in her groin and her legs swelling up in a couple of days. She had received her first shot three weeks earlier. Her imaging revealed three clots. She had no history of clots, took no routine medications, did not travel at length, and was not a smoker. Thus her risks for even one clot were extremely low. She was not asked the date of her shots.

Elderly Man – Stroke, Death

A woman in her 70s told me her husband had his first stroke four days after his second shot. He then had three more strokes while in the hospital, and passed away, less than six weeks later, having never come home from the hospital. She said he was healthier than she was and didn't smoke. I asked if anyone had inquired about the dates of his shots, and she said no one had.

Elderly Woman – Fatigue, Poor Balance, Stroke

An average-weight, very active woman in her 80s complained of fatigue and poor balance since the day after her booster shot. This slowly worsened, and three weeks after the booster, she appeared to have fainted, and family said she was drowsy and very weak for twenty to thirty minutes. She did not want to go to the ER and said she was fine after resting. Two weeks later, she had a few minutes of right-sided weakness, and then another two weeks later, she had persisting right-sided weakness and numbness one day. She went to the ER, where MRI revealed a stroke. There were seven weeks of fatigue and overtly reduced balance, with two neurological events between the booster and the hospitalization for a stroke. Her right leg remains weak, and she still has diminished balance. She was not asked the dates of her shots in the ER.

Elderly Woman – Headaches, Blood Pressure Issues, Microclot Potential

A thin, healthy woman in her 60s received her shots in April and May and her booster about six months later. She complained of a vague headache with mild fatigue that started late in May. She had not had a high ESR, indicating significant inflammation, in her available medical history or knowledge. Upon checking, she had an ESR of 57 in May and 43 in August. In early August, she complained of a headache and vision changes at work one day. This was 11 weeks after her second shot. She went to the ER, where she had a negative brain CT scan. She subsequently had similar episodes in September, October, December, and January, and multiple episodes in February with several emergency room visits. She had another new complaint of tremors in February. She took one medication unrelated to her heart or blood pressure and had stable blood pressure before the health issues in April 2021. Her blood pressure was newly difficult to control. She was seen 19 times between April and December 2021 for her blood pressure issues and various new complaints. I mention more about her problems in later chapters. She also had multiple ER visits, tests, imaging, and a Holter monitor. Extensive workups were negative, and typical causes were ruled out. She was not asked the date of her shots in her ER visits. She still complains of headaches, and she has seen neurology several times. She now takes several medications for her blood pressure and clot prevention. Microclots do not often show up on CT imaging, but I wonder if she had them in her brain.

Elderly Woman – Superficial Thrombus (Clot), Death

A bright, witty, vivacious, thin, and very active woman in her early 90s, who was healthy and took only one prescription for the thyroid and a few vitamins, developed a superficial thrombus (clot) in her right lower leg. She received her shots in mid-February and early March. She stated she woke up with mild pain and swelling in the leg two days after her second shot, which worsened over the next week. The clot was verified by ultrasound. She can also be found in Chapter 4 with Adult Failure to Thrive, which led to her death in 4 $\frac{1}{2}$ months. Before she passed, she was discouraged and angry because she could no longer take care of her home, dogs, 1+ acre yard, cook, bake for others, or drive as she routinely did. She said she had weakened so much, so quickly, and grieved the loss of her vitality. She had had more energy than most 60-year-olds I know.

Elderly Man – Massive Stroke, Death

A frequently smiling, pleasant man in his 70s did have a previous mild stroke many years ago, but he was alert, talked, ate, walked, and had no pain. He was slightly slowed in his response time to talk but otherwise had no long-term stroke effects for the last seven to eight years. He even went to the gym several days a week and exercised with his wife. He was not diabetic or obese and had well-controlled blood pressure. Seven weeks after his second shot, he had a massive stroke that left him bed-bound. His left side was paralyzed, his left arm had severe neuropathy with burning, tingling pain, and he now spoke extremely slow and had a more challenging time talking, was often drowsy, and required a feeding tube as he could no longer swallow. CT imaging confirmed a new stroke. He could not speak well on the day of his stroke, and his wife was not asked the dates of his shots by the ER. He passed away about seven months after another massive stroke, despite therapeutic blood-thinning medications. No one asked about a booster, and I couldn't bring myself to ask his wife about that. I would bet someone counts on us not asking or thinking about it.

Elderly Woman – Pancytopenia, Brain Bleed, Stroke

A feisty, independent, and active woman in her 90s received her shots in January and February. She complained of new-onset memory loss and awful fatigue in late February. In March, she complained of low back and hip pain, causing her to use a walker by April. She developed new pancytopenia in May, a condition in which most or all of your blood count is low. Her white blood cells, the cells that fight infection, went from 5 to 3 to 2.5 as the year went on. Her lymphocytes and granulocytes were also newly low. These are different types of immature white blood cells. Her hemoglobin and hematocrit dropped and continued to decline. In August, she had a hospitalization for hemorrhagic stroke, which means rather than a clot causing a stroke, bleeding in the brain caused it. She received her booster in September. In October, she had much worsened high blood pressure, requiring an ER visit, medication adjustment, and close follow-up. Being in her late nineties and developing so many new health problems so quickly, she and her family chose hospice care. I have seen a half dozen people develop sudden new pancytopenia after their shots, having normal blood counts for years before 2021. I suspect hemolytic anemia; time will tell. Before 2021, I recall perhaps one person with sudden new-onset pancytopenia in nearly five years. So far, we know there is a reduced lymphocyte count in some people after their injections (1) and various hemolytic or blood cell death concerns (2,3).

Elderly Woman – Positional Orthostatic Tachycardia Syndrome (POTS) and TIA

A woman in her 70s complained of new lightheadedness and imbalance nightly since her first shot. She seemed to have a unique sensitivity to position changes, so she was extra cautious when getting up at night and first thing in the morning from a lying position. Eight weeks after her second shot, she had a TIA with weakness and left arm numbness and pain, and a left eye droop. It was resolved during her visit to the emergency room. She did have a history of one TIA in the past, so I considered not including her here. Still, she continues to have sensitivity to position changes a year later, so I decided to include her. Positional orthostatic tachycardia syndrome, or POTS, is a potential side effect of some vaccinations and can cause dizziness upon standing, walking, or position change due to a high heart rate with a drop in blood pressure quickly after the position change (4,5,6,7). Kyle Warner, a professional BMX biker and an athletic young man you will meet later in the book, sadly still suffers from POTS after his shots. I did not see him as a patient, but he tried to share his injuries online and was repeatedly shamed and canceled. A large Facebook group of tens of thousands of injured was also canceled.

Elderly Woman – Pulmonary Embolus

A thin, otherwise healthy but demented woman in her 90s became extremely weak and began often falling less than two weeks after her booster. It is unlikely she knew how to complain of shortness of breath with severe dementia. She was admitted to the hospital, where a large PE was found. She did not have an irregular heartbeat, which is often the cause of clots. A PE is not a typical complication of dementia and she has no history of smoking, so had nearly zero risks for clot formation.

Middle-Aged Man – Pulmonary Embolus, Ventricular Strain

A man in his 60s was obese and sedentary and smoked, which are risk factors for clots. He had no history of heart attack, other clots, recent long trip, or dehydration, which can increase the risk for clots. He was fatigued and mildly short of breath within a week after his second shot. He immediately quit smoking out of fear. He reported a month of gradually worsening fatigue and shortness of breath before going to an urgent care clinic. He was treated for an unconfirmed but suspected pneumonia, and COVID was ruled out. He then went to the ER since he continued slowly worsening a month after the urgent care visit. Upon CT imaging, he was diagnosed with a massive pulmonary embolus. He also had an elevated troponin and an elevated beta-natriuretic peptide (BNP), which loosely but usually indicate some heart damage and heart failure, respectively. His notes reported ventricular strain, which means the heart's lower chambers were strained and somewhat suffered lack of oxygen and, therefore, cell damage. This heart strain can happen from a massive clot in the lung. I asked him if he was asked the dates of his COVID shots while in the urgent care clinic or hospital. He said no, he was not asked the date of his shots. I read the ER notes and inpatient discharge summary, but no dates were documented. The massive clot in his lung was diagnosed 10 weeks after his second shot, yet his symptoms began much sooner. His symptoms started within a week of his second shot. He smoked, so perhaps this was all coincidental, despite the timing. We will never know this side of heaven.

Others – Pulmonary Embolus, Purple Toes/Feet, Petechial Rash, Microclots, Death

A friend of mine works in a medical office. She told me one of their doctors was out of work for a PE in the late summer of 2021.

I have seen an additional 5 people with new-onset complaints of purple toes, feet, and/or fingertips in the last 8 months of 2021. Another half dozen different people complained that their usual tiny or small varicose veins suddenly were swelled larger or were darker in color, which worried them. None of the people who complained of this and showed me their feet or legs for these complaints were unvaccinated. Nailbeds are purple or gray-purple, and sometimes all the toes or the distal feet are purplish in color. A couple of people had toenails become loose, which can happen with a lack of oxygen to the tips of the toes. The feet and ankle veins suddenly bulge out, becoming newly noticeable to some people.

One person had a red-spotted, petechial rash only on the feet and dark purple toes. Both started the day after her COVID shot, followed by intermittent rectal bleeding three weeks later and hospitalization for COVID illness one week later, less than five weeks after her second shot. She passed away at home in hospice shortly after hospital discharge.

Microclots in the feet, legs, liver, intestine, lung, heart, or brain do not show on usual ultrasound imaging. This is why likely thousands have been told that no stroke was seen on CT or MRI despite stroke symptoms. I have had several patients such as this. This is why thousands have been told, I suspect, that no vessel appeared blocked at a level to have caused their chest pain or heart attack. I have had a few patients like this. These are micro clots. D-dimer blood testing can confirm this but must be interpreted with caution and are less reliable for diagnosis in older people. Further, family members told me they had to ask their loved one's doctor to test the D-dimer, or it wouldn't have even been checked. In these cases, variable causes can be ruled out, and the timing of shots with the timing of onset of signs and symptoms can give clues.

I have seen similar dusky purple or gray toenails or fingernails in people very ill, with oxygen dropping in COVID pneumonia, except these people were not ill with COVID and had normal or just slightly dropped oxygen saturation levels and normal vital signs. These people did have the shots and therefore spike protein in their bodies. Of course, low oxygen from any cause can cause purple or blue nailbeds, fingers, and toes, but so can micro clots in tiny capillaries, which are the tiniest blood vessels of the fingers and toes. I saw plenty of dusky purple or gray-blue fingernails in dying or dead patients when I worked in the ICU and ER many years ago. No, I don't normally see purple or dark gray fingers and toes in my current role; it is unusual to regularly see this in primary care. It is also normal to have old people who have had a stroke or blood clot, but nowhere near normal to have this many people with clots in just 8 months. Until 2021. Research supports the formation of various clots after these inoculations (8,9,10,11,12,13).

Natural Immunity

We have no count on how many people would have been spared a life-threatening clot if natural immunity were considered because no one researched this issue. Even if they had, would it have made the evening news? The risk of clots is likely to rise higher with over-stimulation of the immune system, such as in post-COVID illness, recovery, and then followed by vaccination. This was the case for someone in his 20s, whom I know, who developed a PE. He was told the clot in his lung was from his COVID illness a couple of months earlier. The proximity of the shot was much, much closer than that. I have encountered a few people who say they were told their clot was from COVID illness, but they were not asked the dates of their shots which were between the illness and the onset of their clot symptoms. A person in their 20s has an extremely low risk for a clot, even from COVID illness. It could have been the illness, the shots, or combined effects. We may never know this side of heaven. The research will take years. Is anyone even doing this type of research in the young? Will it be announced or canceled if and when the research is done? How can we ever really know an answer if there is not have a control group that has not been given mRNA via injection when the research is done? So if anyone even wanted to know, why did the world insist on people taking an experimental vaccine for that which they were already immune to or whom were needed for a control group?

Spike Protein, Clots & Athletes

Spike protein is spike protein. I don't care how one gets it. It damages endothelial lining (the inner lining of arteries and veins in the body and in the tiny blood vessels inside organs), which creates a cascade of events for increased likelihood of clot development in some people. Clot risks with these shots are elevated and known (14) but usually ignored or denied. Brandon Goodwin, a professional basketball player, hushed by the NBA, had a PE within a month of his shots (15). An ultrasound technician reported seeing clots shortly after the shots in young and otherwise very healthy people. How unusual, the person said, as this just started to happen in 2021. One of them was a woman in her 20s who was an avid runner, thin, and had zero risks of developing a blood clot, just like Brandon, the NBA player. Her massive clot went from her groin to just above the knee.

You will encounter more information about athletes in chapter 3.

Final Thoughts

So far, research and reporting are leaning heavily toward clot promotion and risk. If post-illness clots can be attributed to illness months later, then post-shot clots can be attributed to the shot weeks or months later. The vessel damage is from spike protein; it makes no difference how spike protein was obtained until research proves otherwise. Further, scientists now know that spike protein continues to be produced far beyond just your upper arm where the shot was administered. Spike protein does aggregate in some organs, such as the liver (16), and its effects are found in the brain, heart, lung, ovary, and kidney, as is noted and strongly cautioned by Dr. J.P. Whelan (17) and much research reviewed by Dr. S. Been (18), among others. People have multiple clots after the shots, which is unusual compared to the past (19). In 2021, just one pharmaceutical company's anticoagulant medication saw a 20% operational growth, and that same company saw a 91% increase in operational growth in their bio-similar cancer treatment products (20). Wow, why such a spike in using these medications (no pun intended) in one year?

Further, the same anticoagulant medication will remain one of the top three drugs in sales at least through 2026 (21). The adverse effects rate is unknown, and longitudinal studies are needed (22). I hope those studies have a control group. It has been over 16 months. Where are the autopsy results so we can learn from these new mRNA injections? The first 100-200 people who unexpectedly died shortly after their vaccination should have been autopsied, and the results widely distributed. Perhaps the first 1,000 or 10,000 would be better suited to those wanting a larger sample size.

Chapter 2
PEOPLE WITH NEW ONSET OR HIGHLY
WORSENED HIGH BLOOD PRESSURE

Middle-Aged Man – Diabetic, High Blood Pressure, Stroke & Heart Attack Risk

A diabetic man in his 50s complained to his worksite clinic staff that he didn't feel right during his monitoring period after his booster. They checked his vital signs. He had a critically high blood pressure of 200/110. After the shot, he was watched in the clinic because he had a bad reaction of near-immediate high blood sugar to over 600 mg/dl after his first shot and was seen by the same staff. He was monitored at the clinic and released after 2 hours, despite the blood pressure remaining very high and not feeling right. It had come down slightly but was still 170/100. I saw him two days later, and his blood pressure was still high, at 164/104. I adjusted his blood pressure medication dosing higher to control it. He, of course, required closer and more follow-up. He is at risk for stroke and heart attack and was advised to go to the ER if his blood pressure rises to a certain level or develops symptoms. He can also be found in Chapter 10. I asked him why he got the booster if he had critically high blood sugar that nearly landed him in the hospital from diabetic ketoacidosis. After his first shot, he said it took weeks to settle back to normal blood sugar levels. He said he didn't want to get the shots but had to keep his job, and his employer threatened to fire him, despite knowing what had occurred the first time.

Elderly Man – Elevated Blood Pressure Despite Superb Fitness Level

A healthy man in his 70s developed new high blood pressure less than two weeks after his second COVID shot. He was started on new medication and required follow up. He reported not feeling right, and his readings were 160-180/90-104. He was not over-weight, diabetic, or lazy. He exercised almost every day. He typically ran 120-130s/70-80 for many years before this new hypertension.

Elderly Man – Elevated Blood Pressure Despite Taking Two Low Dose Medications

A thin man in his 70s who had been very stable on two low dose blood pressure medications for many years developed higher read-ings, by 30-40 points, within a couple of days after his booster. He began checking his blood pressure often at home because he just didn't feel right, he said. He required medication dosing adjustment and closer monitoring to control it. His ESR ran anywhere from 8-19 mm/hr for a couple of years. After his shot, his ESR was newly elevated to 35 mm/hr indicating more inflammation in his body. He can also be found as one of the examples in the liver enzymes chap-ter, chapter 9.

Elderly Woman – Aggressive Medication Adjustments Required

A normal-weight woman in her 80s who had already taken one blood pressure medication complained of not feeling well and reported newly elevated, critically high blood pressures two days after her second shot. Her daughter monitored her blood pressure at home, which went from her usual well controlled 130-140s/70-80s to 180-200/90-100. She required aggressive medication adjustments, including two new medications with escalating dosing and increased follow-up monitoring. She remains on the latest and higher doses of medicine now, nearly a year later.

Elderly Man – Chest Pain and Pressure, Left Arm Pain, Heart Failure, Respiratory Failure

An overweight man in his 80s who had a usual normal blood pressure of 110-130 systolic/70-80 diastolic and did not take any blood pressure or heart medications presented to the office with intermittent chest pain and pressure and left arm pain that started on day 4 after his first shot. His blood pressure was elevated to 182/90, and he had certain ST segment elevation changes on his EKG, which can mean a lack of oxygen or a possible heart attack. His symptoms were relieved with nitroglycerin and aspirin given by the ambulance crew on the way to the ER. Troponin T, an enzyme that indicates heart muscle cell damage, was checked once and was 15.0 ng/L which is normal in a male for troponin. His baseline Troponin T a year earlier was much less. It was 0.01. As nitroglycerin lowered his blood pressure and resolved his chest and arm pain, the troponin would typically have been rechecked over time with an evaluation of trend, mindful of the onset of pain. Still, it was not rechecked before he left the ER that day. For those of you in the medical field who want to blame his kidneys, we cannot because he had entirely normal kidney function before, during, and after this time. His cardiac stress testing was negative for heart vessel disease a few days later. He required a closer follow-up and a cardiologist. He was not asked the dates of his shots recorded in the ER record or by the cardiologist.

He is also the first person in the next chapter, chapter 3. He can also be found in chapters 5 and chapter 13. He was in the ER and had 17 office visits in the year. Then, he had two hospitalizations after his booster.

Update: nearing the end of writing this book, he has been seen with 13 new health problems since his booster. The worst is heart failure and respiratory failure, requiring oxygen 24 hours a day. His prognosis is poor.

Elderly Woman – Increased Dosing for Blood Pressure

A woman in her 70s who took one blood pressure medication experienced higher blood pressure readings in the 160-170s/90-100, less than two weeks after her second shot, which was 30-40 points higher than usual. She knew she didn't feel quite right, she said. This problem persisted, soon requiring an increased strength in her medicine to reduce her blood pressure to its usual range of 120-140/70-80.

Middle Aged Man – Body Pain, Very High Blood Pressure

A previously healthy man in his 60s developed widespread body pain and high blood pressure less than two weeks after his second shot. His hs-CRP was very high, at 35, and his ESR was also newly elevated. Before this time, he had normal ESRs, no pain, and normal blood pressure. He took no prescription medications, instead only vitamins before this happened.

Final Thoughts

Do high blood pressure problems occur in primary care? Of course, they do, and it is expected, but the proximity here is quite close, and the sheer number of people with new or worsened blood pressure is a certain safety signal. ***This safety signal would easily be missed if no one ever asked the dates of a person's shots and the dates they began having symptoms.*** And that is likely what occurred worldwide as hospitals and urgent care clinics were overwhelmed in 2021. Reports will not be made if dates are not asked and timing is not investigated. Remember that very high blood pressures, such as 180/100 or higher, can sometimes lead to strokes. Remember that elevated blood pressures sometimes occur without the person feeling anything. Still, other times can cause a person to have symptoms, such as headaches, heaviness in the chest, and vague feelings of being unwell. I did not include all the patients I had with high blood pressure. It is, of course, common in primary care. I scrutinized several other cases and decided not to include them here when other potential causes or contributors were found. Still, we will never know this side of heaven whether those possible causes or the shot effects increased their blood pressure. I can tell you for certain that the number of young people with high blood pressure and heart rates since their boosters is absolutely shocking. I am crushed in sadness for the young men who were physically fit, don't smoke, exercised regularly, and normally wouldn't be developing high blood pressure or heart concerns for another two to three, or four, decades. Remember, the people I share here did *not* have the COVID illness. Again, the sheer number of people with new or worsened ***high blood pressure and new elevated heart rates is astonishingly increased*** compared with previous years. These shots are certainly associated with cardiovascular changes (1,2,3,4,5).

Chapter 3

PEOPLE WITH NEW ONSET OR SYMPTOMATICALLY WORSENED CHEST PAIN, ATRIAL FIBRILLATION, HEART VALVE FAILURE, HEART FAILURE & HEART ATTACKS

Elderly Man – Chapter 2, Worsened Symptoms

The same man in chapter 2, with the blood pressure escalation and chest pain on day 4 after his second shot, had shortness of breath, palpitations, and chest discomfort again five to six weeks later. He was then diagnosed with atrial fibrillation requiring daily blood thinner medication. He was now on three new drugs. Later in the year, he went back for his booster.

He can also be found in Chapter 5 and Chapter 13 to discuss his further health declines.

Middle Aged Man – Heart Attack

A thin and active man in his 50s had a mild to moderate aortic valve heart problem but no history of coronary artery disease, irregular heart rhythm, or clots, experienced a heart attack 9 days after his second shot. He complained of mild shortness of breath the day after the shot that slowly worsened until he developed chest pain and went to the hospital. He was discharged home after two days. He had another massive heart attack one week later, 16 days after the second shot. There were *no* diseased heart vessels found to explain his heart attack, so he required no stent or bypass surgery. He spent weeks in two hospitals and was placed on a heart transplant list. I have never seen such high cardiac enzymes in all my decades in the field. I have no idea how he is alive but for the grace of God. His Troponin I, an indicator of cardiac muscle cell damage, was over 4,000! A Troponin I of 100 would have been considered terribly high in the good old days! Normal is near 0.04-0.39. His heart valve problem was also worsened by the damage. He hopes to get a new heart. There was no documentation of the dates of his shots in his ER or hospital records. He stated that no doctor asked him the dates of his shots. When I showed him the dates of his shot and heart attacks, he cried out loud and thanked me profusely. I was crushed for days. He is thankfully getting better, slowly.

Elderly Man – Irregular Heart Beats, Chest Pain, Dizziness

A man in his 70s with known atrial fibrillation presented urgently to me asking for an EKG and complaining of dizziness, weakness, and shortness of breath on exertion. He stated he couldn't walk too far or he would get too dizzy. His breathing became more challenging. This was less than household distances and could occur at just 20 feet. His oxygen levels remained normal, but his heart rate was too fast. This had happened the last 3 days and was getting worse, and he admitted slight intermittent chest pain now, too, if he exerted himself. He got his booster 4 days ago. His EKG revealed his usual atrial fibrillation, but the rate was much too fast, called rapid ventricular response. He said he was fine and had no symptoms at all if he rested in the chair or laid down. But if he exerted himself with normal walking room to room, his heart raced irregularly, causing his symptoms. He had had atrial fibrillation for years, and it was well controlled with medicine, and he lived an enjoyable retired life, including frequent golfing.

A cardiology visit was arranged in less than 72 hours, and he was given strict guidance on when to call 911 over the weekend if he had chest pain or started to have symptoms at rest. He stated he would rest all weekend and wait for his cardiologist. He was fearful of the hospital as it was so unusually busy, he said and refused to go to the ER. As I looked back at his record, I found he had been in the ER for chest pain and dizziness a week after his second shot over 6 months ago. I asked him why he got a booster if he ended up in the ER less than a week after that shot, and he said he didn't even think of it then, and no one else had asked him the dates of his shots.

As I was trying to wrap up and end the visit, he shared that his old high school friend had just passed from a heart attack and had taken his booster a couple of days prior. He kept talking and shared that his current, athletic, slender, and healthy friend, who took no medicine and had no medical history, had a massive heart attack one week after his booster. He stated this friend had been in the heart hospital for a month, now had only 13% of his heart pump (ejection fraction or EF), and that the doctors told him if he hadn't been so very healthy, to begin with, he would have died. At least they acknowledged the cause in that man, but no one knows if it was reported to the antiquated Vaccine Adverse Event Reporting System (VAERS).I didn't ask this man if he knew anyone else who suffered heart problems shortly after the shots. He simply volunteered the information to me after I asked him the date of his shot.

Elderly Man – Worsened Heart Failure, and Hospice

A man in his 80s had heart failure. He was active, did yard work, drove, and was fully independent. He would have been classified as stage 1 New York Heart Failure, the mildest and easily controlled stage. He was stable, and with rare, minor medication adjustments over the years, he was treated outpatient and had no hospitalizations for heart failure. Less than a week after his second injection in March, he complained of terrible fatigue and loss of ability to do his usual activities. He simply had no energy and became short of breath too quickly with any exertion. He was soon hospitalized for worsened heart failure, and his EF dropped down to 14% in April 2021. His EF was 40% in late 2020. This sudden 26 percent drop in his EF explained his shortness of breath, lack of energy, weakness, and fatigue. He required his son to move in with him as he could no longer care for himself. He was soon after referred to hospice.

He can also be found in chapter 15.

Elderly Man – Heart Attack, Death

A man in his 70s received his second shot in mid-March and passed away less than three weeks later, in early April. His wife reported he passed from a heart attack. She said he had been upset and was grieving the loss of his father who was in his 90s, and who had just suddenly passed away.

~

Final Thoughts

If cardiac catheterization reveals clean coronary arteries, meaning that no 'blockage' could be identified as the cause of chest pain and an acute heart attack, but the laboratory Troponin levels, indicating heart muscle damage, were very elevated in some cases, we must work-up for myocarditis and other cardiac injuries. I have seen this several times recently, as many people's hospital records have a listed diagnosis of elevated troponin levels among their myriad of other reasons for their recent hospital stay.

Do the events I shared in this chapter occur in people anyway? Of course, they do. But the proximity of the injection to the event is suspect. It is more than enough to raise a safety signal. Why would the FDA and CDC choose to lightly dismiss heart conditions when they were listed in their own worklist in *October 2020* (1)? Heart complications have been seen, including heart attacks and failure (2,3,4,5). We are warned to expect more myocarditis, pericarditis, and the risk versus benefit decision should be done more carefully for the young, especially children(6).

Chapter 4
PEOPLE WITH NEW ONSET FAILURE TO THRIVE AND/OR ENCEPHALOPATHY

Elderly Man – Fatigue, Weight loss, Failure to Thrive

The wife of an 80-year-old man complained that he became very fatigued and passive the day after his second shot. I did not ask for his shot dates, she volunteered them to me. He began sleeping about 4 more hours per day than he used to. He would sleep in later, doze after breakfast, and had to take a long nap every afternoon. She would sometimes have to wake him at mealtime. He was losing weight, and they didn't know why. He seemed mildly confused and was frequently drowsy. He rarely drank a beer and never took Tylenol but had new-onset elevated liver enzymes in his lab results. Liver enzymes were newly elevated one month after his second shot. His alkaline phosphatase was 189 IU/L, ALT/SGPT was 66 IU/L, and GGT was 275 IU/L. Those lab results had been normal for years before now. His alk phosphatase ran 89-98, his ALT was 9-16, and his GGT ranged from 12-16 in the prior years. His urine, blood count, thyroid hormones, chemistries, and other labs were normal. Cranial nerves were intact, and strength was equal bilaterally. He hardly spoke, didn't volunteer any conversation, gave short, straightforward answers to her attempts to talk, and then would sit quietly again or fall asleep. He complained of being unsteady, and the farther he walked, the more unsteady he became.

His wife said they lived a very full life, were always active, never napped, and enjoyed each other and their frequent outings before his shots. She was angry as their lives had drastically changed, and she complained he "just sits there" and barely spoke or interacted anymore. They declined CT imaging as they did not want to go to any medical facilities, and his wife was convinced it was from the shot. I reduced some of his medications downward in dosing due to his fatigue, liver enzymes, and weight loss leading to lower blood pressure with a high risk of falling, referred him to physical therapy and neurology, and encouraged him and his wife to work on improving his fluid and food intake. He perked up a bit after lowered medications and some time. Primary care cancer screenings were negative. His liver enzymes did return to normal after 6 months, and he gained a couple of pounds back, but his overall mental status was still nowhere near his usual functioning.

Increased sleep and fatigue, reduced appetite, unintended weight loss, significantly reduced mobility and talking, or increased weakness are signs of adult failure to thrive in an end-stage disease or illness, such as severe, end-stage dementia or Parkinson's disease. This man had no signs or symptoms like he and his wife had reported before receiving his second shot. This could also be partly hepatic encephalopathy from the elevated liver enzymes, but his mental status and symptoms persisted, though lessened, even when they returned to normal levels. I can hear folks now saying he just had dementia. Dementia doesn't just drastically change a person in one or two days. It happens over time. I suspect he had micro-clots in the brain, causing encephalopathy. Micro-clots are microscopic fragments of the size of a typical clot that would show a stroke on a CT scan and won't be seen on imaging.

Elderly Woman from Chapter 1 – Unusual Fatigue, Failure to Thrive, Nausea, Death

In her early 90s, the witty woman previously mentioned in Chapter 1 with the superficial clot in her leg complained of awful fatigue and lack of usual energy, sleeping more, unintended weight loss from reduced appetite, and intermittent nausea. These began very mildly within a week of her second shot but worsened over time. She eventually required medication for nausea to get any food down and chose hospice a few months later. She passed 4 1/2 months after her shots. I suspect micro-clots to the intestine and/or brain. She was tested on more than one occasion and did not have the COVID illness. She only had the shots. I have had three other people with complaints of intermittent but frequent nausea since their shots. I didn't even have to ask them. They came right out and said they were mildly nauseous every day ever since their shots and that their stomach just wasn't the same, and had they had slowly begun to lose weight and were much more fatigued because of it. GI workups availed no reason or relief. I have had two of the people with abdominal complaints with positive D-dimers, indicating a higher probability of clot formation.

Elderly Woman – Fatigue, Cough, Congestion, Pneumonia, Weight loss, Blood Pressure issues, Ear Ringing

A woman in her 70s got fatigued and weak the day of her second shot. The weakness persisted, and she fell four times in the two weeks between her second shot and her office visit. She also complained of terrible ear ringing and trouble hearing beginning a week after the shot. She started losing weight and was sleeping longer than usual. Her family said she was less talkative. Three weeks after her second shot, she developed a cough and congestion. One week after that, which was one month since her second shot, she was admitted to the hospital for pneumonia and suspected

COVID. Her COVID test was negative, and she was treated for pneumonia. She unintentionally lost 25 pounds in the six months after her shot. Eventually, she recovered from all this and took her booster. Less than two weeks after her booster, her home health nurse notified me of consistently higher blood pressure readings, and her daughter had also found higher readings. Her systolic blood pressure was now 150-170s, whereas it used to run 130-140s. Her blood pressure medications had to be increased. She has lost another 5 pounds and has worked with physical therapy several times to keep her ability to walk. She can hardly hear at all now and still complains of ear ringing.

Middle Aged Woman – Fatigue, Joint Pain, Acid Reflux, Abdominal Pain, Bowel Movement Changes, Heart Palpitations, Brain Fog

A normal weight woman in her 50s complained of terrible fatigue, joint pain, acid reflux, abdominal pain, changes in bowel movements, palpitations, nearly passed out and visited the ER, and got 'brain fog,' which she felt slowed her down at work and made her go to sleep earlier at night. She lost a few pounds without trying. In two months, she had all these new problems that first began 2-3 days after her booster shot. In previous years, she visited one or two times all year. In the last 5 months since her booster, she visited primary care 5 times and had an ER visit and an urgent care clinic visit. No one asked her the dates of her shots except me.

Elderly Woman – Lack of Energy, Fatigue, Memory Issues, Unkempt, Rambling Speech

An overweight woman in her 70s complained of a terrible lack of energy, significantly increased fatigue and sleep hours per day, and memory concerns that began one week after her shot. She went from being very well-groomed and articulate to being unkempt and often rambling in her speech, and she reported this was caused by the lack of energy to intently and caringly groom and dress well and a loss of clarity of thought. She had unchanged labs except for the ESR, which went from 29 mm/hr to 58 mm/hr. Her symptoms persist still. Again, usual diseases are fairly easily ruled out with screenings, labs, imaging, and consultants if needed.

Elderly Man – Heart Failure, Hospice, Mental Status Change, Death

A man in his 90s with heart failure on hospice was alert and oriented and often played cards. He played solitaire and card games with his family. He spoke at length of his long and exciting life the last time I saw him before his status changed. He did require intermittent nitroglycerin and oxygen for chest pain about once a month, and some medication changes intermittently to keep him stable and comfortable with his heart failure. His daughter reported that he passed out and fell less than 3 hours after his second injection. That was the last time he would walk. He could no longer stand on his own nor walk at all. She stated his mental status had also changed. He had been confused since, with intermittent agitation and some hallucinations. The family had to take shifts to keep him calm and safe. He began refusing solid food after just a couple of bites. He was treated for a possible presumed urinary tract infection (UTI), which can sometimes cause these confusion symptoms in a frail elder. That made no difference at all. Thus it was unlikely a UTI. He spent the last weeks of his life not knowing his family members and acting like a different man. He passed 3 weeks after his second injection.

Elderly Woman – Fatigue, Confusion, UTI, Death

A woman in her 80s received her first shot in springtime and became very fatigued with new confusion the next day. About two weeks later, she was treated for a urinary tract infection (UTI) and remained fatigued and mildly, but pleasantly, confused. Her labs revealed an ESR of 83, which is very high inflammation, and alkaline phosphatase, a liver enzyme, of 179 was also newly higher than normal. All prior ESR labs and liver enzymes were normal. She did not have a history of recurring urine infections. One week after she had recovered from the UTI and repeat urine samples were normal, she received her second shot. Within a few days, her mental status declined again. She rarely spoke, rarely ate, and wouldn't drink. She was newly agitated if awakened and wouldn't stay awake long. She went to the hospital because she wouldn't eat or drink and slept too often, and passed within a couple of weeks. I suspect micro-clots in the brain and liver. Others will attribute her demise to urine infection and blame sepsis, except she never had sepsis or required hospitalization for the UTI

Elderly Man – Weight Loss, Fatigue, Hospice

Another man in his 90s unintentionally lost 17 pounds in 5 months after his first shot. He also slept an average of 4 more hours per day. He was admitted to hospice in 6 months. Cancer and thyroid problems, which can cause unintended weight loss or gain, were ruled out.

Elderly Man – Fatigue, Less Talkative, Walking Issues, Weight Loss, Mental Decline

A man in his 70s with Parkinson's disease is brought by the family who reports he is sleeping more hours per day, being less talkative, having trouble walking, eating less, and losing weight. Now, these are normal in end-stage Parkinson's. The problem is, these concerns began less than 2 weeks after his shots, and before his shots, he wasn't in end-stage disease or even near it. All of these symptoms started at the same time were of sudden onset, and before this time, he could walk safely and get himself out of bed daily. He also talked with his family and ate at each meal. Typically, the downward mental status and physical deterioration in Parkinson's are gradual, barring a trigger ill health event. This case is much harder to determine, but the timing is reasonably suspect and the acute changes are of concern. Typical causes, such as a urinary infection, flu, pneumonia, and COVID illness, were ruled out.

Elderly Man – Fatigue, Mental Decline, Body Pain

Another man in his 70s complained of moderate to severe fatigue since his first shot. It was bad enough to prevent him from going back to get his second shot. I did not see him near this time, nor did I advise him to avoid his second shot. I saw him, and he told me this story himself months afterward. He also complained of his memory not being nearly as sharp, which started with fatigue. His ESR was 12 in 2019.

After his shots in 2021, it was 32, then 45 three months later. He did not gain weight, change his diet, or start smoking or drinking more to contribute to a rise in his inflammatory marker. He had no pain complaints in 2019-2020. In 2021, he complained of the low back, hip, knee, and heel pain. He said he was seeing several other specialists for his pain complaints.

∾

Final Thoughts

The complaints of new, severe fatigue, significantly reduced energy, and unintended weight loss was seen in at least three dozen people over the age of 65 between March-November 2021. Most of them, except the man on hospice – because labs are typically not checked when someone is on hospice- had elevated ESR, liver enzymes, or both. Some of them were worked up for cancer, which was negative. Things can be, and were, ruled out. Checking the dates of shots and the onset of symptoms can be a clue. I am not sure why I need to type out that last sentence about checking dates and the start of symptoms. I have found very, very few emergency room encounter notes or hospital admission or discharge notes, and I read them nearly daily, that listed the dates of someone's shots before a new stroke, clot, heart attack, passing out, pain flare, confusion, etc., etc. I have seen very few, but not all, ER or admission notes mention 'COVID shots x2' or 'COVID vaccinated and boosted' or 'unvacci-nated.' I love emergency room personnel. I used to be an emergency room nurse in a primary heart hospital many years ago and loved it. I can guarantee that ER doctors and nurses do not have time to report vaccine reactions, even if they suspect one. Further, we cannot find what we never look for.

Does failure to thrive occur in elders of advanced age? Yes, it does, but this is a huge number of failure to thrive patients of various ages for this concise window of time for just one provider! I suspect neuroinflammation or micro-clots in the brain, causing encephalo-malacias and encephalopathies. In other words, softening or scar-ring the brain and brain damage. This might look like a quick onset of dementia, which is not typical of dementia. Usually, dementia takes years to develop. Another massive safety signal. Who cares enough to deeply study the elderly, mainly because they are the people this entire campaign was supposed to protect? Perhaps Norway does (1). Neuroinflammation, inflammation of the brain and/or nerves, has been found after these inoculations (2). I suspect millions see their doctors and specialists trying to find answers.

There are also reports of acute confusion or hyperactive encephalopathy post-vaccination (3,4,5). I have had at least a dozen patients suspect for this adverse effect. They and their family reported a change in temperament that was strange and unusual for them, with brand new anxiety, panicky feelings, insomnia, and restlessness. We will never know this side of heaven. I doubt these encephalopathies will be studied in great detail because they can be caused by various things, including drug and vaccine reactions. In 2022, I am seeing it in the young men and women after their booster. This problem will be tough to sift through and determine with the elderly and is too easily attributed to old age. Ageism, age discrimination, is alive and well.

Chapter 5
PEOPLE WITH NEW ONSET PAIN OR PAIN FLARE-UPS

Gasoline on One Flame of Inflammation

This section is so challenging. In my opinion, it is gasoline on one flame of inflammation. There are too many people to discuss, and many of their complaints and situations would be repetitive and redundant. I estimate I have seen at least 150 people with either new-onset pain or old injury or surgery site pain flares. So I am summing them up. ESRs in many of these people ranged from a normal 2 to 13 in previous years and from 45 to 93 in 2021 after their injections. Now I can hear some people say that many things can cause the ESR to rise, so there is no way to prove it was the shots. These could be poor diet changes, weight gain, smoking onset, severe arthritis, severe allergies, illness, or injury. I agree, and that is true. These people didn't have any common culprits, and work-ups for usual and potential causes were ruled out. The only thing they had different in 2021 was new shots.

Several people had very old injuries, even decades ago, with zero or just slight pain for many years, but now suddenly, in 2021, after injections, they complained of heightened pain. People who had occasional, mild low back or hip pain now complained of severe, in some cases excruciating, and totally debilitating pain. Many had ER visits and new orthopedic, physical therapy, and pain management referrals. People who had joint replacements with zero pain for years since the joint replacement now had pain at a replaced joint. Many had no pain but now had face, ear, scalp, neck, shoulder, or hand pain. Many people had new-onset heel pain. A few report a feeling of awful cramps all over or spasms that can come and go with no rhyme or reason. One woman, who you'll encounter again in Chapter 12, had widespread pain with a condition that can damage the kidneys and threaten life. I have a friend whose family member developed severe joint pains right after his booster, which became excruciating when he tried to walk and was nearly para-lyzed. He was told by his doctors it is autoimmune related. I suspect spinal nerve inflammation and, in some cases, transverse myelitis for some of these people, which is further discussed in several upcoming chapters. These were all different people, suddenly experiencing a severe pain crisis to get them to seek medical care. This is a massive spike in unusual pain cases in 9 months, from March to December 2021. Gasoline on one old flame of inflammation and, in some instances, neuroinflammation. This is another reason why emer-gency rooms and urgent care clinics were overwhelmed in 2021. Who exactly is studying this phenomenon?

$\backsim$

Final Thoughts

Do we see these issues routinely? Yes, of course, people are seen for various complaints of pain, but not these types of problems. No, not decades-old injuries that hadn't caused pain in decades suddenly flare 'out of the blue' with no apparent reinjury or cause but just flare within days to weeks after their injections. No, not pain in total joint replacements. Not a dozen people complain of facial, toe, or heel pain in just a few months (1). No, not facial, scalp, and ear pain frequently. No, not sudden onset inexplicably sudden and intolerable low back pain and/or hip pain. No, not daily. No, not when imaging or Xrays are entirely unchanged from years ago, but pain at the site has badly flared. But if suddenly your one old, minor problem area, a smoldering flame, or one flame of bodily inflammation has gasoline poured on it, it will hurt much more.

The same man you read about in chapter 2 with blood pressure problems and chest pain and chapter 3 with new atrial fibrillation and heart failure experienced much pain after his booster. In 4 months, he frequented medical care and the ER and had a hospitalization, with many specialists now on his case. His ESR went from 4mm/hr in the summer to 49 mm/hr the month after his booster in early fall and remained at 48 mm/hr two months later despite several courses of prednisone. He often complained of new scalp pain, headaches, ear pain on and off, neck pain, leg pain, back pain on and off, hip pain on and off, and pain in the balls of his feet and in his old knee replacements. He only had occasional, mild back pain in 2019 and 2020. He was diagnosed with temporal arteritis, among other things.

One woman had surgery behind her ear, cutting a nerve that caused persistent, intolerable pain. The surgery successfully relieved the pain that started a week after her injection.

I know of a young woman who had cervical spine surgery in hopes of alleviating her neck and shoulder pain, and her pain remains unrelieved.

I have had, or personally known, many people with negative workups, and normal or unchanged xray, CT, or MRI imaging to explain their strange new or much worsened pain problem. Some are absolutely surprised to learn their imaging came back normal. Some say "If it is normal, why do I have so much pain?". I predict it may be gasoline on your one flame of inflammation, or the trigger on your immune system. Injury to the nerves, especially the spinal cord, can be devastating. This leads me to the next chapter.

Chapter 6

PEOPLE WHO SAY "IT FEELS LIKE MY LEGS AREN'T THERE" OR "IT FEELS LIKE MY LEGS ARE DISCONNECTED FROM MY BRAIN AND WON'T WORK" OR WHO HAVE UNUSUAL NEUROLOGICAL SYMPTOMS

Elderly Woman – Frequent Falling

A woman in her 50s complained of frequently falling since her booster. She had not had a history of falling. She stated her legs just give out all the time now.

Elderly Woman – Low Back Pain, Trouble Walking

A woman in her 70s complained of terrible low back pain that wrapped around her left hip at times and trouble walking. She said, *"it feels like my legs.. aren't there."* According to her, the onset of this problem occurred less than a month after her second shot and lasted a few months. Thankfully, her issues resolved after a long course of prednisone, a steroid.

Elderly Woman – Tremors, Trouble Walking

Another woman in her 70s complained of notable tremors and that intermittently, her legs just wouldn't cooperate with her to get up and walk. She reported concentrating and taking extra time to get up and walk, and it was difficult and shaky. She stated it felt like her insides were tremoring, but it couldn't be seen. Her family sometimes saw tremors in her hands, arms, head, and upper body, but the patient complained she felt tremors all the time and all over her body for months. She also stated her taste and smell were altered. She did not have COVID and was not ill in any other way. I did not need to ask her when this started. She told me this problem had started *within a couple days* of her second shot, and she knew this because it was the same day *her husband* had received his second shot. Thankfully, these issues resolved on their own after a couple of months. She shared more news with me and said her previously healthy husband, who *"was healthier than me"*, and took no medications, didn't smoke, and was very active, *passed from pericarditis and a heart attack three weeks after his second shot.* Her symptoms began after her shot and well before he died, so her tremoring was **not anxiety** from losing her husband.

Elderly Woman – Fatigue, Absent Leg Feeling, Low Back Pain

A woman in her 80s said she was *quite fatigued and that it strangely felt like her legs weren't there,* she had low back pain too, and these complaints began less than two weeks after her shots. She *fell and broke her hip* less than a month after her booster.

Elderly Man – Legs Felt Disconnected, Fatigue, Altered Taste & Smell, Nerve Damage

A lean and spry man in his 90s complained, *"it feels like my legs are disconnected from my brain and won't work."* His symptoms of this problem and generally feeling moderate fatigue and depleted energy levels began *less than a month* after his shots. He also complained of altered taste and smell. He unintentionally lost 16 lbs in 2021. *He did*

not have COVID and was not ill in any other way throughout the year. He was
tested by neurology and was told he had myelin damage in the
nerves of his legs after electromyography testing. He was told it was
"chronic demyelination" of the nerves. The onset was sudden and
his life devastatingly changed in less than a months time... that is
not 'chronic'! In my opinion, it is dismissal and denial of reality
toward an old man, and it is wrong.

Myelin, in simple terms, is a layer of your nerves that transmits
messages between the brain down the nerves and to the muscles to
function and move. He is discouraged now and exhausted all the
time. He is contemplating MRIs to rule out transverse myelitis,
which may occur after Covid inoculations (1,2,3). Multiple sclerosis
can newly occur and flare after COVID vaccination (2,4,5). There is
much more research to support this discussion. I have only included
a few of the numerous studies on nervous system involvement.

Elderly Man – Altered Taste & Smell

A man in his 60s complained of altered taste and smell after his
shots and new shoulder pain. He was tested negative for COVID
and had no other symptoms. Three other people who were not ill
with COVID tell me their taste and smell have been altered or
nearly gone since their shots. Loss of smell and taste could be
damage to cranial nerves I and VII, respectively.

Final Thoughts

Transverse myelitis can cause extremely weakened legs, near-
paralysis at the low spine, and bladder and bowel incontinence. In
straightforward terms, transverse myelitis is inflammation of the
spinal cord that extends across the width of the spine, especially at a

certain level. That level determines which part of the body a person has trouble using and where the function is lost. It is sometimes improved with early Prednisone, and sometimes it is not. I listened to the testimony of a surgeon who suffered from transverse myelitis after his shots and who had to retire very early. He couldn't stand long enough to do surgery anymore. He said he would have had another 15 years as an orthopedic surgeon. Before putting him in this book, I tried to contact him out of respect but was unsuccessful. Since he shared his testimony on video, I think he would be okay with me mentioning him here.

Speaking of physicians doesn't really fit in this chapter, but I must share as the above surgeon's story reminded me of an unusual phenomenon. Never in all my years have I had so many patients tell me that their specialty doctor passed away suddenly and unexpectedly. No, it wasn't COVID, they'd said, but they didn't know why because it was so sudden, and the last time they had seen their doctor, they looked fine. I admit most doctors do not share with their patients when they are sick. Still, in 29 years, perhaps four or five patients shared a story like this. In the last six months, I have heard five similar stories.

Observations, especially of trends, and the asking of questions form the basis of scientific inquiry. May we honor people, and 'science', by inquiring, not dismissing.

Chapter 7
PEOPLE WHO FALL AND BREAK BONES (FRACTURES)

Many individuals have fallen and broken bones. A fracture is a broken or cracked bone. I am not an orthopedic provider. During six months, there were three pelvic and two hip fractures, a clavicle fracture, a humerus (upper arm) fracture, a wrist fracture, two lumbar spine fractures, and an ankle fracture just for one provider.

Yes, elders fall sometimes, and we see follow-ups from fractures. No, we do not see this escalated incidence of fractures in a usual year, just in 2021. Others have noticed, too, including a radiology technician who agrees that fractures have skyrocketed. We shall see if it continues through 2022.

Is this from pain issues in the back, hip, and legs causing weakness and falls? Is this from neurological changes like myelitis, neuropathies, or clots to the brain causing a person to be severely weak, lightheaded, or imbalanced and then collapse and therefore have a sudden, hard fall breaking a bone? Or is this from bone density changes quickly predisposing people to osteoporosis?

Science will take many years to figure this out. I'm going with neurological and pain issues, but it's just an educated guess. As one coworker said, "What's with all these fractures?" Who exactly is studying the increased rates of falls and fractures? No research is available on this particular topic yet.

A woman in her 80s received her first injection. She has her first episode of unexplained passing out, known as fainting, or syncope, less than a week afterward. She collapses and the fall causes a fracture in her lumbar spine or hip. No one asks if or when she received her shots. I will share a typical scenario here because it would be repetitive, but this one woman represents a dozen people. Are we to ignore old people because this is wrongly assumed 'normal' for old people, even when they had never passed out or fallen before and led active abundant lives?

~

Final Thought

One more typical scenario is heard. The person reports a mechanical fall, doing something they have always done safely before. But this time, they didn't perceive risk or react in time to the dangers and fell. Simple accidents happen. Now, this is common when someone falls and happens in fall scenarios, but why the escalation in 2021? Why didn't they perceive the risk or react in time? Why did so many people report this in just 9 months?

Chapter 8
PEOPLE WITH NEW ONSET BLADDER AND BOWEL INCONTINENCE OR BLOODY BOWEL MOVEMENTS

Middle-Aged — Weakness, Bladder and Bowel Incontinence, Weight Loss, Death

A middle-aged man with sickle cell anemia complained of increased weakness, causing him to be recently wheelchair-bound and the sudden new inability to control his bladder and bowel. He had multiple specialty providers. He reported he had been unintentionally losing weight, had no appetite, and put up with this incontinence for over a month. None of his consultant providers could tell him why. The symptoms all began the same month as his shots. He passed away in a few months. I suspect he suffered from transverse myelitis, explaining his severe weakness, inability to walk, and bladder and bowel control loss.

Elderly Woman – Bladder and Bowel Incontinence

A woman in her 70s complained of sudden onset of the loss of urinary and bowel control within a month of her injections. Some may say this is common for older women. This is unusual that both would occur so suddenly and precisely simultaneously, especially in a woman who didn't even have a leaky bladder with sneezing and coughing before this new-onset complaint.

Observation – Bloody, Loose Bowel Movements

I have seen at least five people who had one bloody, loose bowel movement, and then the bowels returned to being brown in color the next time they moved them. This typically occurred within 3-6 weeks of the shot. They did not have a history or a sign of hemorrhoids or even constipation. They did not have any positive work up when they agreed to them. Does this happen in primary care? Yes, it does, occasionally. Not five people in six months telling the same story of one frightening, bloody bowel movement.

Final Thoughts

MRI of the spine can reveal signals of transverse myelitis. Transverse myelitis has been found after critical COVID illness and after the shots. There was a noted "extremely high" rate in the clinical trials(1). Perhaps that is why the FDA said transverse myelitis in October 2020 is a projected side effect(2). Why wasn't this listed on the product insert, and why weren't you told about this potential side effect as part of informed consent before taking your experimental shot? It is not likely you could have read it on the product insert, like thousands do daily when they get prescribed a new medication. You couldn't have read it on the insert, because it was blank in 2021. This fact was just one more 'first' for 2021.

What were you told at your 'informed consent'? I asked dozens of people if they were informed that these inoculations were not studied nor FDA approved in the usual fashion, and 90% of them said no, they were not told. I asked dozens if they were informed of the different and new shot types compared to all other vaccines in their lifetime, and 100% said no. I asked some if they were told that outcomes were supposed to be under research and were scheduled to be studied on the public until 2023, and again, they all said no.

Chapter 9
PEOPLE WITH HIGH LIVER ENZYMES

Elderly Man from Chapter 4 – High Liver Enzymes

We return to the older gentleman in his 80s who you met in Chapter 4 here. Liver enzymes were normal-looking back two years before his month of injections. Afterward, they were abnormally high, and they remained higher than normal for six months. I have seen several more people with transiently elevated liver enzymes, lasting from 3 to 12 months.

Lab Examples

A few examples of lab results from people with various liver enzyme elevations after their shots include the following:

Person 1 GGT 30-60 for two years before to 163 after shots and 209 still a year later.

Person 2 ALT 15-20 IU/L before to 72 after, and though the GGT was still normal, it was 13-15 before and 48 after the second shot.

Person 3 GGT 30-46 IU/L before to 66 after the second shot, then 106 after the booster.

Person 4 ALT 13 IU/L before to 125 after the second shot.

Elderly Man – Abdominal Discomfort, Excessive Bleeding, Elevated Liver Enzymes, Bile Duct Stone, Heart Attack, and Kidney Damage

A man in his 80s developed upper abdominal discomfort. He didn't want to use the word, *pain*, one week after his second shot. Older folks can be very stoic. Especially older, retired military men. He usually had alkaline phosphatase 49-117 IU/L in his history, the month after his shots, it elevated to 243 and then 465 IU/L. His AST/SGOT was usually 9-17IU/L, and it elevated to 44, then 61 IU/L. His bilirubin was 0.3-0.8mg/dl, and after his second shot, it escalated to 3.8 mg/dl. His GGT went from 17-35 IU/L to 168 the month after his shots, to 570, 924, 653, and more recently, is down to 273. He did not drink alcohol, a common cause of an elevated GGT. His albumin, a type of protein, is newly low. He had an endoscopy, a scope placed down his esophagus into his stomach and upper abdominal organs to check for bleeding. This occurred less than a month after his second shot. He had another endoscopy two weeks later for the same problem, despite usually effective medication. He had an ER visit for a nosebleed three months later. He was not on a blood thinner or medication that could cause bleeding. He did have a history of an arterial-venous (AV) malformation in his stomach that hadn't caused a problem since the beginning of 2019. He had a third endoscopy during hospitalization for bleeding five months after the first one. Several clots and a stone in his bile duct were found, which had no doubt contributed to the elevated liver enzymes. One month later, he was again hospitalized for severe bleeding and had another endoscopy. The bleeding was so intense that he suffered a heart attack and kidney damage. All this bleeding was from AV malformation, and his liver issues were from the bile duct stone, but was the shot the trigger? Or a contributor? Was it gasoline on one flame of inflammation on his previously asymptomatic and smaller bile duct stone? Did he have a sub-clinical level of gallbladder or bile duct inflammation that escalated from gasoline on one flame of inflammation? His pain began one week after his second shot. His liver enzymes were never elevated before. Why did he have a nosebleed? Why did he keep re-bleeding worse and worse despite proper treatment and when it hadn't bled or required treatment in over two years? Seven months, four endoscopies, and recurrent bleeding. He is now frail and weak. I debated with myself whether to include him in this book. Still, I decided to do so because of the proximity of the onset of his symptoms, including pain, because his liver enzymes were never elevated before his shots, and because I have had several people with escalated liver enzymes and bleeding issues after the shots. There is a ton of coincidence or there is a ton of correlation. How much causation there is will likely remain unanswered.

Elderly Man – Fluid Build Up, High Blood Pressure, Pulmonary Hypertension

A man in his 60s received the shots in May and June. The new heart and stomach doctors did not give any explanation or disease as a cause of the extensive fluid build-up in his stomach, which is called ascites. Hepatitis, cirrhosis, liver failure, cancer, and heart failure were ruled out. His liver enzymes were not elevated. His ESR was 44 in June and 57 in October, and 71 in February. His health continues to decline. He was recently diagnosed with high blood pressure in the lungs, called pulmonary hypertension

Final Thoughts

I had three other people with a nosebleed or coughing up blood that started one to three days after their shots. One of them was on a blood thinner for over a year and had never had bleeding before. Yes, I have nosebleeds occasionally in primary care. But not this many in just a couple of months, in early 2021. They occurred 1-3 days after their shot, so I felt it was worthy of being noted.

Spike protein is found in the liver and the human genome after vaccination(1). Still, the mainstream repeatedly announces these shots don't have anything to do with your genes. The average person doesn't read or critique research nor have time to search beyond the news narrative. Research has discussed mesenteric and hepatic vein clots, in other words, clots in your gut or intestine or the veins in and on the surface of your liver (2), which can cause abdominal pain, poor appetite, nausea, fatigue, and lethargy, as well as bleeding. Some clots can be post-shot autoimmune responses(3) or bring about liver inflammation and hepatitis (4,5,6,7). Episodes of bleeding, as well, have been seen after these shots (8), sometimes which lead to new or flared immune-related kidney diagnoses (9,10,11).

Chapter 10
PEOPLE WITH SUDDEN UNCONTROLLED BLOOD SUGAR OR DIABETIC KETOACIDOSIS

Middle-Aged Man from Chapter 2

We return to the middle-aged diabetic man in Chapter 2 now. He stated he was kept at the clinic longer for monitoring seven months earlier because his blood sugar escalated to over 600 within a few minutes of receiving his injection. He reported that he didn't feel right, so they checked his vital signs and blood sugar. It took several weeks for his blood sugar to return to normal.

Elderly Woman – Diabetic Ketoacidosis

For the first time in her life, a woman in her 80s was hospitalized for over a week with diabetic ketoacidosis (DKA), a critical illness. This hospitalization occurred less than 2 weeks after her booster. She was a type I diabetic.

Elderly Man – Erratic Blood Sugar Levels

A responsible man in his 60s complained that his sugars were newly and strangely erratic, sometimes high and sometimes low, immediately after his injection. He had to check his sugar several times a

day for feelings of high and low sugars and dose his insulin accord-
ingly. He had always kept his diabetes very well controlled, and
followed sliding scale insulin dosing several times a day. This lasted
nearly a month, and then his blood sugar began to settle down to his
usual well-controlled levels.

Elderly Man – Kidney Failure

A man in his 70s received his shots in April and May. His diabetes
has been well controlled for the last several years. His lab test that
determines how well controlled the diabetes is, called the HbA1c,
jumped up two points to becoming uncontrolled 2 ½ months after
his shots. After his booster, it jumped up another point, becoming
more uncontrolled, despite the new diabetic medications that were
added, and increase in dose six months earlier. Further, his kidney
function suddenly declined from normal filtration and creatinine
before his shots to stage 4 kidney failure after his second shot. His
creatinine went to 3.26, and his filtration rate dropped to 16. He
had normal kidney function for years before this. Thankfully, he is
steadily improving from the worsened diabetes and kidney trouble,
with close follow up, adjustment of several medications, and some
tincture of time.

~

Final Thoughts

Before receiving these injections, people with poorly controlled
diabetes have a less effective immune response to these new biologic
agents (1), meaning the shots for these people may not be helping
them avoid infection as well as someone without diabetes. But these
people had immediate drastic changes in their blood sugar levels
after their shots. Did this also hinder their immune response? We
don't know. Since diabetics are at a higher risk of critical illness
from COVID, were diabetics included in any clinical trials? I could

be wrong, but I don't remember that being addressed in Pfizer's clinical trial before US vaccinations started. Because diabetics are at a higher risk for infection in general, and uncontrolled sugars place them at an even higher risk for disease, could this have actually been detrimental to their ability to fight any infection, including a COVID 'breakthrough' infection? Some astute diabetics already know that this inoculation raises, at least temporarily, their blood glucose and changes several laboratory results (2).

Since we are on the subject of blood laboratory results and changes, I am reminded of a scathing post from a physician I once read. He mocked and accused the other doctor who shared his views of not knowing anything about COVID's critical illness and how he had never seen how thick the blood of dying COVID patients is. He spouted his hard work in trying to save people in ICUs with this never before seen thick blood. I'm sure he was stressed out, and I feel for him. Still, I don't work in a hospital anymore, but I regularly see this crazy thick blood in my patients in primary care who have been vaccinated. The lab techs commented on it quickly after the vaccines were rolled out. They are negative for COVID, they just have an old-fashioned upper respiratory infection that seems harsher and more complicated to fight off, with a heavy positive cold agglutinin test, or they are just getting their routine labs drawn. Blood viscosity rises can indicate and contribute to various health concerns and are common in metabolic syndrome, and are also seen post-COVID vaccination (3).

Chapter 11

PEOPLE WITH FREQUENT AND HEAVY MENSTRUATION OR MISSED CYCLES

Menstruation Changes

A woman in her 30s presented to me with two heavier and longer than usual menses one month after her injection. Her periods were now twice a month and lasted 7 days, but they used to be 5 days. She passed clots directly, which was uncommon for her. It was now the second month, and she again had bleeding in two weeks. She stated she had had typical 5-day, once monthly cycles her whole life until now.

A post-menopausal coworker complained of strangely returned and frequent cycles, bleeding every two weeks, which began nearly two weeks after her injection. A cycle occurred every two weeks for almost six months, then reduced to monthly, and persists. She is contemplating a work-up for the post-menopausal bleeding, which could be a symptom of endometrial cancer.

A salesperson complained of heavy and more extended periods. She was stunned to hear that other women experienced this same problem after their shots. She asked me why this wasn't in the news.

An acquaintance of mine shared they had heavier periods with a few small clots since taking the shots.

A young woman in the medical field reported no periods three months after her second shot, then a normal period. After the booster, it stopped again for three months, then resumed.

Another woman I know who works in the medical field reported some women just won't stop bleeding. She estimated she had seen at least twenty women. She shared that her coworkers had also seen dozens of women with the same problem. These medical professionals are involved in the work up and monitoring the issue.

Final Thoughts

I don't go looking for much of these issues. Many people share their problems with me without any depth of inquiry. The first three women in this chapter shared this with me on the same day. What are the chances? Why are women still, in 2021, being dismissed, mocked, and disbelieved by doctors, patriarchal corporate organizations, government that is supposedly all about empowering women, and the media? I once read a significant group page on one of the social media sites about women sharing their side effects, but I can no longer find it. I admit I don't read or seek much GYN related research because I am not an OB/GYN provider and never preferred this area of medicine or nursing. Still, this group of physicians and their proof more than suffices to explain the hiding of women's issues and related problems (1). The coming years will tell us even more.

Chapter 12
A WOMAN WITH SEVERE RHABDOMYOLYSIS (MUSCLE BREAKDOWN/MUSCLE WASTING)

A woman in her 70s presented with new-onset pain in her joints and muscles all over her body. She said the worst pain was in her hands, wrists, and forearms. The pain, though, was all over. Her arms, legs, knees, and feet hurt as well. The onset was subtle less than one week after her second injection and gradually worsened over the next few weeks. The pain had been increasingly mounting for those weeks, and she said she couldn't take it anymore. She said she thought about, but resisted, going to the emergency room twice because the pain was so bad a few days and nights in a row, just before I saw her. She was afraid to go to the hospital.

After seeing her critically high creatine kinase (CK) lab, I thought about sending her to the emergency room. Creatine kinase indicates a person's muscle breakdown rate, which we all have but which should be within a specific range. It can change depending on our exercise, overexertion, such as severe muscle strain in weightlifting, or other various health insults to the muscles. The kidneys are at significant risk of failure when this happens. I treated her to improve her condition and alleviate her fears of going to the hospital. I had her push as much water and fluids as she could handle, used alternating NSAIDS, Tylenol, and topicals to the most painful places, and after getting her labs, gave her prednisone. Her normal CK levels went from 74-96 U/L before, for years, to 1,256 U/L after her shots.

Two weeks later, the CK level was 943, which is still critical. Then after another six weeks, it was 247, which is still higher than normal. Six months later, her CK returned to a normal level and was 70. Throughout the Rhabdomyolysis (severe muscle breakdown, often causing pain and no doubt the cause of her pain), she unintentionally lost 20 lbs in 3 months from the severe and uncontrolled muscle wasting. Her appearance drastically changed. She was not overweight when this problem began. She was fearful as she couldn't understand why she was losing so much weight. She looked thinner and frailer each time I saw her, every couple of weeks until she was better. She thankfully recovered with frequent evaluation and treatment. She is now nearly back to her baseline weight before injections.

This woman's ESR went from 13 mm/hr in 2020 to 47 two weeks after her COVID shots. Her liver enzymes were also transiently elevated after the shots, running 13-24 for two years and then elevating to 125-132 IU/L before returning to her normal baseline. Her high sensitivity C-reactive protein, a cardiac event risk marker, was 0.8 in 2020 and elevated to 8.74 after the shots in 2021. Her calcium did the same, usually running 9 mg/dl and rising to 12, then returning to baseline after three more months.

∼

Final Thoughts

I have seen a dozen other people with elevated calcium after their injections. Some of them have elevated potassium levels as well.

Initially, their kidney function is unchanged, but later after several months, a few have had declines in kidney function requiring closer monitoring and in some cases, medication adjustments.

Rhabdomyolysis has been noted after these injections (1,2) and arthritis and myalgias (3).

Chapter 13
A WOMAN WITH VOCAL CORD PARALYSIS AND A MAN WITH BELLS PALSY

Elderly Woman – Vocal Cord Paralysis

A retired woman in her 60s who is allergic to many things, and carries an Epinephrine (EPI) pen because of her allergic risks, took only her first injection. In about 36 hours, she began to have a sore throat and hoarse voice. Her throat became quite painful with talking within a few days, and she began losing her voice. She entirely lost her voice, and the effort to speak just one word was excruciating for about a month. Trouble speaking after just a few minutes persisted for three months, so she went to see her ENT provider. The ENT doctor informed her and documented in consultation, which I reviewed that she had left vocal cord paralysis likely from the injection. The woman had to meet with a Speech Therapist for vocal cord exercises, which she still practices intermittently and independently. She still reports that if she talks at length for nearly 20 minutes on the phone, her voice will still fade out, requiring her to get off the phone and rest it. At follow-up, the woman told me that her ENT doctor told her he had seen several others with the same reaction and that he had seen several ear and throat effects from the injections. I believed her because she was a nurse in her younger years and didn't tend to exaggerate her conversations, and I had seen several ear complaints as well.

Middle-Aged Man – Bells Palsy

A friend of mine has a male family member in his 50s who got Bells Palsy within two days after his first shot. Later in the year, less than two weeks after his booster, he had significant and worsening pain in his legs and needed a walker. A neurologist worked him up and confirmed it was an adverse reaction from the shot. Soon after, he needed a wheelchair, which he still uses most days.

Final Thoughts

After these shots, many neurological issues have been found (1,2,3,4,5,6), too many to list. Neuroinflammation can create facial and other weakness, twitches, tremors, seizures, pain, trouble using certain parts of the body, depending on which part of the brain or spinal nerves are affected, and vision and hearing changes, among other issues.

Chapter 14
WOMEN HIGHLY SUSPECT FOR ALLERGIC PURPURA RASH (ALLERGIC VASCULITIS)

Elderly Woman – Body Pain, Rash, Diarrhea

A woman in her 70s complained of generalized, whole body pain and upset stomach with diarrhea for several days before developing a red, raised spotted rash on her stomach, back, upper arms, thighs, and buttock. The rash began as red spots, then turned purple-brown and sometimes black. As the lesions turned darker in color, they began to itch fiercely. She reported the itch was terrible, kept her up at night, and was often painful when she did scratch though she tried not to. Topical steroid cream did not help the rash. She had not started any new medications to trigger allergic vasculitis, but she had received a COVID booster shot less than two weeks before her symptoms began. I did not have to ask her the date of her shots, she volunteered them saying she had not felt right since. Allergic purpura or allergic vasculitis can be characterized by this type of rash and typically has pre-rash, whole body, or systemic symptoms such as whole-body pain and upset stomach. This condition is usually caused by a drug reaction, though it can be caused by a virus or bacteria or autoimmune disorder, which was ruled out. She reported a similar rash after her earlier COVID shots, but the initial rash was barely noticeable and not problematic or itchy then. Thankfully, she responded reasonably well to steroid treatment and allergy medication. There was no kidney involvement. Her ESR was 54, elevated from her usual and normal range. She had to be treated with two courses of prednisone and she remained on an allergy medication months later.

Elderly Woman – Chills, Sweating, Joint Pain, Nausea, Diarrhea, Rash

A woman in her 60s complained of intermittent chills and then sweating with severe joint pain for about a week before she developed this same type of rash as the previous lady. Her symptoms started within two weeks of her second shot. She, nearly tearful, complained the itch was terrible, and she couldn't sleep for days. She also complained of a poor appetite and some nausea and diarrhea intermittently for days. She had not started any new medications, and viral, bacterial, and autoimmune illnesses, including COVID, were ruled out. Her ESR went from 2-6 over the last two years to 25 after her booster. Her platelets, which are cells that help your blood clot, were abnormally elevated by nearly 150 points from her baseline. Platelets had gone from 268,000 to 340,000 over the last 2 years to 451,000 after her booster. She also responded to steroids and allergy medication, though it took her a longer duration of treatment and more follow-up visits to improve.

Elderly Woman – Rash, Fatigue, Stomach Pain, Joint Pain

A woman in her 80s complained of a rash on her arms, legs, low back, abdomen, and buttock. I did not have to ask her the dates of her shots. She volunteered the information stating it started within a week of her booster. She complained to me that she saw a dermatologist three times from whom she tried topical medications with no relief. The rash started with some days of fatigue, upset stomach, and joint pain, with slightly raised or flat red spots soon following. The joint pain subsided, and the rash spread. The spots would enlarge and then turn dark purple-brown and itch. She doubted she would get a skin biopsy from the dermatologist, and she was miserable and didn't want to wait for another dermatology appointment, so I treated her. She had been dealing with the rash for two and a half months before seeing her. It was my third suspected case of allergic purpura. I gave her prednisone. She was happy.

Middle-age Woman – Rash, Stomach Pain, Joint Pain

A woman in her 60s who works in the medical field developed a low-grade fever, widespread joint pain, mild stomach upset, and this rash less than two weeks after her booster. She had it on her chest, abdomen, buttocks, and legs. It lasted four months. She also told me that she had a friend with the same type of rash, which occurred after her booster.

Final Thoughts

Allergic purpura, sometimes called systemic vasculitis, typically affects children after a virus, bacterial infection, or drug or substance reaction. In children, usually, it tends to resolve on its own. Thankfully, none of these ladies suffered kidney or other organ damage when I saw them, which can occur in vasculitis. Vascul- means the vascular system, or vessels and the inside of all organs since they contain vessels, and -itis means inflammation. This is usually a rare condition in children (1). But it was in adults in the past year, and I suspect it wasn't rare. I had precisely zero cases in my previous five years of clinical primary care practice. In my previous 29 years as an RN, I had seen this rash two or three times when working in a critical care unit with very sick people on many medications. Allergic vasculitis is usually preceded by a prodrome illness of fever, aches, and/or upset stomach with diarrhea, and has been seen after this vaccination (2,3,4,5). Other rashes, especially shingles, have also flared or been newly encountered post-COVID vaccination (6,7,8). I believe I have had three post-vaccination shingles cases.

Chapter 15
PEOPLE WITH TINNITUS (EAR RINGING OR SOUND) AND EYE COMPLAINTS

Elderly Man – Tinnitus

A man in his 60s complained of terrible loud tinnitus that began in September 2021, shortly after his booster earlier that same month. In 2019 and 2020, his ESR went up and down within normal limits of 8-27 mm/hr. A couple weeks after his booster, his ESR was 68, indicating much inflammation. In December, it was still 59, and his complaint persisted. The ear ringing is still present today. He has seen several specialists with no relief.

Elderly Man – Tinnitus, Limited Hearing

A man in his 80s complained of awful tinnitus since the day of his booster that severely limited his hearing and ability to communicate. He was getting very frustrated and withdrawn as no one could help him.

Elderly Man – Vision Loss

The man in his 80s with multiple new health problems was mentioned in four previous chapters. He now has heart failure and requires oxygen. He developed pain in his head around his ear, and then right-sided vision loss and was diagnosed with temporal arteritis less than two months after his booster.

Elderly Woman – Tinnitus, Ocular Migraine, Vision Changes

A woman in her 70s complained of mild tinnitus for years and a rare ocular migraine a few times a year. An ocular migraine causes a vision change and headache. After her booster, her tinnitus worsened, becoming constantly bothersome, and her ocular migraines averaged 1-2 times a week.

Elderly Woman – Eye Pain, Blood Clots

A woman in her 60s is seeing the eye doctor for a possible clot in the back of her eye and bilateral eye pain since her booster. She tells me her sister recently had the booster as well and just had surgery for four clots in her stents in her legs despite being on medication to thin the blood. She shares that she is the primary caregiver for her sister, who is younger than she is but frail and cannot live alone. Before she leaves, she tells me that the vascular surgeon who operated on her sister told her that he is now seeing clots in teenagers.

Final Thoughts

I have seen two other people with complaints of constant, loud ear ringing or intermittent shooting pains in or around the ear or on one side of the head and neck that started within a few weeks of injection. One of them was the man in his 90s with heart failure from chapter 3. I have also seen four people with unusual vision changes within a few weeks of their injection, which have needed the care of an eye doctor. Her eye doctor told one woman that nothing could be done for her vision loss. It was some sort of optic neuritis or inflammation of the optic nerve. Another woman was told she had glaucoma and was treated for it for six months in 2021. She didn't notice any improvements, and then at her follow-up appointment, she was told by the eye doctor he wasn't really sure what it was but that her vision loss wasn't glaucoma after all. She said he had no answer for her and no definite diagnosis. I wonder if he asked her the date of her shots and the date of the onset of her symptoms or did an MRI. I have read about some eye and vision changes and diagnoses post-vaccination (1,2,3). Tinnitus was actually discussed on an evening news outlet. It was mentioned as being a very rare and mild side effect.

Chapter 16
PEOPLE WHOSE CANCER WORSENED, WERE NEWLY DIAGNOSED WITH CANCER, OR HAD LYMPH NODE SWELLING

Elderly Woman – Breast Cancer

A woman in her 70s had a lumpectomy with radiation and chemotherapy eight years ago. She had a normal mammogram in September. She had a booster in November. She felt a lump in January. I sent her for a diagnostic mammogram, and she has a return of breast cancer.

Middle-Aged Man – Cancer, Death

A man in his 40s received his first shot in September. He began coughing up blood in late October. He was diagnosed with lung cancer in December. He had a plan with oncology to start chemotherapy in February. He passed before treatment could be started. Of course, cancer could have been there a while, and the timing could be purely coincidental. We will never know. I don't like the fact that I have seen a half dozen people with nosebleeds or one or two episodes of coughing up blood post these shots, I've never seen that after any other type of vaccine.

Elderly Woman – Large, Hard Lymph Nodes

A woman in her 80s who had been receiving regular chemotherapy for lymphoma had been doing well and feeling well. She was independent and active. Since receiving chemotherapy, she had shrunk and softened lymph nodes in her neck. The neck nodes were the only ones that were ever enlarged before, and she had been responding very well to her cancer treatment. She developed new-onset large and hard lymph node swelling in her groins less than two weeks after her booster. She had never had any other node swelling nor enlarged groin lymph nodes before and had been undergoing chemotherapy treatment for months when this happened.

Elderly Woman – Cancer

A woman in her 80s who had a history of a colon resection for a rectal tumor had been doing well, living life without health concerns, and was without any routine medications. It had been over a year since her surgery and she had since returned to living her normal life. Her cancer returned in her liver in August, less than two months after she took the shots.

Elderly Woman – Hysterectomy

A woman in her 70s received her shots in March and mid-April. Near the end of April, she started having an unusual vaginal discharge. She was diagnosed with endometrial adenocarcinoma in June and had a hysterectomy.

Elderly Woman – Endometrial Cancer

Another woman in her 60s had a total hysterectomy for endometrial cancer diagnosis in 2021. She was diagnosed 5 months after her injections, and I don't know when her symptoms started. These two women were not overweight and had a normal body mass index. Yes, I would have seen 1-2 women in a year with post-menopausal bleeding, but they are typically obese women. I have sent six additional postmenopausal women to gynecology for further workup of vaginal bleeding or unusual vulvar changes this past year, which easily surpasses the previous 4 years.

Elderly Man – Unusual PSA

A man in his 80s had a usual PSA of 2.3-2.8 for the last several years. In 2021, two months after his shots, it was 6.5.

~

Final Thoughts

I had three women who felt a thick, swelled area in their breast between two and three months after their shots who had lymph node or lymph chain swelling.

Typically, I would refer about one man per year to urology for possible prostate cancer in a year. Still, in mid to late 2021, I referred three men for newly elevated prostate-specific antigens (PSA) in six months. Typically, I would refer one to two women for an ultrasound or biopsy evaluation of a lump or mass on an abnormal mammogram in a year, but I have referred eight from mid-2021 to early 2022. This occurred even though I followed the new guidance to delay mammograms at least six weeks after a woman received COVID shots due to possible local lymph node swelling (1). Thankfully, most of these people returned with benign lymph node swelling, benign cysts, or inflamed scar tissue and just lived with the minor discomfort, inconvenience, and fear until answers were identified. I don't know if they would have had these issues whether or not they would have received the injections. I do know that lymph nodes, cysts, prostates, and scar tissue, among other parts of the body, can swell and enlarge in the setting of high inflammation. I also know that Dr. Cole, an expert pathologist, has recently been warning of an increased occurrence of some fast-growing, unusual masses and cancers (2). He is not alone, as some military physicians, with their lawyers, have also warned of an exponential increase in cancers (3). Researchers also note a 394% increase in armpit lymph node swelling compared to the last two years (4). Lymph node swelling now requires closer follow-up and careful scrutiny of diagnosis (5,6,7). The spike protein is associated with increased cancer pathogenesis (8,9,10).

I know three people who had their cancer return and two newly diagnosed outside of work.

The simplest definition of cancer is abnormal cell division. High levels of inflammation can lead to abnormal cell characteristics, and if this persists or progresses, it can lead to abnormal cell division. A simple way to think of this is skin cancer. When skin is overexposed, the sun can severely inflame skin cells. Another simple way to think of this is esophagus or stomach cancer. Chronic alcohol use or many years of chronic unhealthy dietary intake cause situations that inflame the esophagus or stomach lining, and then cancer can develop. A third simple way to think of this is lung cancer from years of smoking, which inflames the various structures in the airways and lungs. Finally, obesity is well known to be a state of chronic inflammation, which is a significant reason why obese individuals have a higher risk of many cancers, including cancers of the thyroid, esophagus, liver, gallbladder, kidney, pancreas, colon, rectum, breast, ovary, uterus, and cervix (11). This has been widely known in medical literature for many years. Why weren't there strong media campaigns to reduce junk calories and promote weight loss to help prevent life-threatening cancers? After all, cancer has been a leading cause of death for many years. Why doesn't life-threatening cancer from obesity scare people like COVID does? Good question. Why didn't the government invest billions into obesity prevention and treatment like it invested in COVID shots? Those are subjects of another book.

Chapter 17
A YOUNG MAN WITH CHEST PAIN
UPON A NATURAL VALSALVA

Natural Valsalva Maneuver

If you held your nose and kept your mouth closed while attempting to exhale or pop your ears after an airplane flight, or if you ever squeezed your stomach muscles and held your breath to deliver a baby or relieve constipation, you were doing a Valsalva maneuver. A natural Valsalva occurs whenever a normal or exertional bodily movement creates pressure in the chest and abdomen. A healthy person tolerates a natural Valsalva without issue.

Young Man – Chest Pain

In his early thirties, a healthy and thin man with no psychiatric history or recent unusual stressors received his second shot. One evening, he was sitting on the floor about 2 weeks later, bent forward, pushed himself up off the floor, and developed crushing chest pain. He stated he felt heavy pain in his chest and thought he might die from the pain and weakness. He felt his arms and legs get weak and numb as well. His chest pain persisted. His friend drove him to an urgent care clinic, where he was told he had anxiety and a panic attack. No labs were drawn, and one electrocardiogram (EKG) was done. He was given medication for anxiety. A few days later, the chest pain and symptoms returned when he was at rest. He went to the emergency room, where he was told he had anxiety and a panic attack. No labs were drawn, and one EKG was done. It was normal. He was sent home with medication for anxiety to take once daily. At either of these encounters, no one asked him if and when he had the new shots. No one ordered simple lab work to ensure his safety. No one checked his heart sounds or comfort levels in different lying positions, which can offer important clues sometimes.

It is entirely possible he simply had anxiety. It is possible he had an unusual vagus nerve response from the Valsalva that creates a momentary drop in blood pressure, though that does not typically cause severe chest pain. Instead, a drop in blood pressure would cause dizziness and/or tunnel vision and could be postural ortho-static tachycardia syndrome (POTS). It is possible that he had a mild case of myocarditis, but lab work and other test inquiries were not made.

Young Male Athlete – Myocarditis, POTS, Reactive Arthritis

A previous young athlete in his late 20s, and professional mountain biker, Kyle Warner, was dismissed and suffered *multiple misdiagnoses of anxiety at different hospitals* before his deeper workup and diagnosis of Myocarditis, POTS, and Reactive Arthritis. He is now unable to ride his bike and regularly sees a cardiologist. You can read about him and thousands of others at Kyle Warner, Professional Mountain Biker (realnotrare.com).

Final Thoughts

The European Soccer Association has seen a high escalation in myocarditis, heart attacks, and deaths in 2021. This caused France to stop giving the vaccine to those *under 30* and Singapore to warn their players not to exercise for two weeks after getting the shot (1). Post-vaccination myocarditis has been reported and generally affects the young (2,3). Researchers call out policymakers for caution related to myocarditis rates in children (4). Researchers plainly state that long-term post-vaccination myocarditis effects are unknown and call for extensive studies of children(5). Why is the US now pushing to inoculate small children and infants? Denmark comments on how inadequate our reporting system is and that the US reports lower rates of myocarditis than they have found (6). NCAA golfer John Stokes has suffered a season and possible career ending myocarditis side effect four days after his shot. He warns he knows of other athletes who have suffered the same, on a TikTok (7).

To sum this up, we have higher than usual rates of myocarditis, myocarditis being mistaken for anxiety in some cases, researchers calling for caution and larger, long-term study of post-vaccination children, and known under-reporting of side effects including adverse events of myopericarditis, lasting heart damage in some cases, and more death with this new shot than all other vaccines in our lifetime, combined. We also have censoring, mocking, and canceling of the injured, many scientists, and doctors who diagnose, study, and treat them.

I have asked a few pediatricians what the rate of post-COVID illness myocarditis in children is, and they do not respond. I often read research abstracts and articles that insist the benefit outweighs the risk of heart issues in the young. Still, I have yet to see this rate comparison, and when I refer to their cited studies of support, very few childhood ages are actually addressed. You know, you must read data, not just abstracts. Results or conclusions paragraphs and abstracts often dismiss actual data results in tables and study outcomes. You will never see this unless you read studies thoroughly and can critique real data numbers and ascertain their context, or change your sources of information. In sum, an article abstract, write up from a journalist, or the evening news edition may state one outcome, but the evidence of the research and references clearly lack support for it. Still, it becomes a loudly repeated narrative. Worse, it becomes a societal push without thought for you or your children's health or life.

Myocarditis risk is referenced dozens of times in https://www.saveusnow.org.uk/COVID-vaccine-scientific-proof-lethal. Yes, many of these discuss a very small risk, and that benefit outweighs the risk. Even they repeat the narrative of 'mild' and 'rare'. They were not mild for Kyle, John, or Brandon. They are not mild for the young men seen often in 2022. How many of us have read of a young person suddenly dying recently? Many in their sleep. Or, perhaps, depending on your feed, you see none because they were canceled. You must read referenced material at the end of an article or research paper in many cases because statements are made broadly but not about pertinent age groups being discussed, or cite another 'news' agencies statement. That is not research or reality, it is parroted narrative. Keep in mind that age group risks from the vaccine are not addressed directly, and if anyone can find an actual rate of post-COVID illness myocarditis in those under 30 or in children, do share.

How can a pediatrician recommend these shots to masses of children without knowing actual rate comparisons or being able or willing to discuss them? How can a pediatrician simply parrot the CDC narratives and pressure parents and kids without considering actual lives of whom they are supposed to be protecting, helping grow up healthy and strong, and healing?

Chapter 18
ISOLATED AND BED-BOUND PEOPLE WHO GOT SICK RIGHT AFTER THEIR CAREGIVER GOT A BOOSTER BUT THEY DID NOT GET A BOOSTER

A bed-bound man with severe dementia and no other health problems in his 70s was suddenly eating less, losing weight, sleeping more, and occasionally coughing. His oxygen was dropping to the mid-80s when I saw him. He is bed-bound and has one full-time paid aide and one family member who cares for him. He didn't leave the tiny apartment and saw no one else except his nurse and me once every 8 weeks. The man received his first two shots many months ago. He did not get his booster shot as it is hard to get him out of his room, but the aide told me his family member did get a booster just under two weeks before the man got ill. The family member was not sick. The demented man was treated for pneumonia, suspected COVID at home, and recovered. These symptoms are consistent with COVID or pneumonia in a frail elder.

A bed-bound woman with severe dementia in her 90s was suddenly breathing faster, sleeping more, occasionally coughing, and having trouble tolerating her tube feeding. Her oxygen was dropping to the low 80s when I saw her. She had not vomited, but the food stayed in her stomach longer than usual, so the feeding rate was then lowered to toleration. She sees no one else except her full-time caregiver, whom she lives with. The family is taking extra precautions due to COVID fears, so they had not been visiting for over six months. She had her first two shots many months ago but did not receive her booster, as it was hard to get her out of the house. Her caregiver, who was not ill, received her booster 2 weeks earlier. The frail, demented woman was treated for pneumonia, suspected COVID at home, and recovered.

An isolated, obese woman in her 60s told me she got sick and recovered from COVID. She sought no medical treatment. She asked me how that could have happened, both how she got COVID illness and how she survived. She had been terrified. She told me she never left the house in nearly two years, never saw anyone, worked on her computer, called and zoomed people, got groceries delivered, wiped them off, and skipped all the birthdays and holidays to prevent getting COVID. The only time she ever left the house in nearly two years was to get her COVID shots.

~

Final Thoughts

What are the odds? I am not a statistician. The encounters in this chapter occurred the same day. *Viral **shedding** is when a person gets a biologic type of vaccine or gene therapy, leading to microscopic virus particles in their nose or mouth that can potentially be **spread to others***. It occurs most abundantly and often the first 10-14 days after receiving the substance (1). Because it can potentially spread to, infect, and affect others, the government created guidance, *in 2015*, on when and how it should be studied with certain types of gene therapy or biologic agents (1). **Viral shedding is found in the airways and nasal swabs of those inoculated with these new COVID 'vaccinations'** (2,3). Some researchers admit it is unknown how long the viral shedding may occur (3). It makes sense then that one eye doctor's office I know of did not want any patients entering the building for at least 14 days after a patient had received the new COVID shots. What has been done if the newly vaccinated actually spread the COVID virus? What has been done if the newly vaccinated spread viral particles that created unknown health effects in others? We will not know for years and perhaps not ever know. The pharmaceutical companies did not research this issue to my knowledge, and they still haven't, unless I am mistaken. If anyone has that particular aspect of research concerning these new vaccines, please do share it. Perhaps it is in the pages of unreleased Pfizer documents. I don't know. I did read their released research upon the EUA, and among other lacking qualities, it was not mentioned.

Chapter 19
PEOPLE WHO SAY THEY HAVE BEEN "SICK EVER SINCE"

Elderly Man – Sick Ever Since

A man in his 70s complained of terrible fatigue that started the next day after his shot. I did not have to ask him anything. He volunteered all of this information to me. Within three days of the shot, he got headaches, neck, shoulder, and back pain, swelling and pain on one side of his mouth and cheek, altered smell and taste, and a strange sensation that something was stuck in his eye. The eye sensation passed after three more days. He was not ill, nor was his family, and many things were ruled out. He was angry he couldn't do his usual lengthy walking outside due to his new fatigue and pain. I gave him prednisone mainly due to the mouth swelling and pain. When he returned to follow up, the headaches, mouth complaints, and smell and taste issues were resolved, the fatigue was lessened but not gone, and his neck and back pain, though lessened overall, persisted and really flared up if he walked over a mile. I extended a lower dose course of prednisone as he requested, and his pain symptoms resolved. He still complains, many months later, of moderate fatigue compared to before his shot.

Elderly Woman – Constant Allergy Symptoms, Fatigue, Low Energy

A woman in her 60s arrived in what I call 'omicron week.' I went outside to see her in her car since she was a suspected case. She complained of a fever, body aches, congestion, slight cough, and worsened fatigue. She had COVID, and I treated her, and she recovered at home. While explaining her current condition and symptoms, she also said she felt sick and fatigued ever since she had the shots, but she felt even worse now that she had COVID. She described having constant allergy symptoms, congestion, fatigue, and very low energy since her second shot. She described sleeping more and longer and having trouble doing her usual daily activity due to fatigue, and this was before she got omicron illness.

Middle-Aged Woman – Sick Ever Since

A woman in her 50s told me that she received one shot in February 2021 and had been "sick ever since." She has a long history of multiple environmental and medication allergies and carries an EPI pen. She said her old friend, a doctor, was upset she had the shot knowing of her many allergies. The woman complained of recurrent 'sinus' and 'upper respiratory' infections for nearly a year, requiring urgent care center visits for them. She also had fibromyalgia in the past, which she overcame with significant lifestyle and diet changes, exercise, and various nonpharmacological pain control measures. Her fibromyalgia symptoms recurred within two days of her first shot and lasted a month but did pass. A side note about fibromyalgia: as recently as 2017, a local medical school still taught its students that fibromyalgia is an entirely psychological issue. How do I know this was still taught? A physician assistant student who attended there told me so during our clinical time together. What a shame, considering there are volumes of books written by physicians on the matter, and the American College of

Rheumatology and The Journal of the American Board of Family Practice recognize it (1). It seems most things conventional medicine doesn't have an answer for, know how to treat, or don't make a profit from are often, and still, labeled as psychiatric issues. It seems to me they are mostly minorities', women's, or children's issues.

Elderly Woman – Respiratory Failure, Breast Pain

A woman in her 60s who had known mild pulmonary fibrosis developed respiratory failure within one week of her second shot and was hospitalized. She has required an increase in her routine medications since. She has also had repeated upper respiratory infections since, something she did not have before this time. She also complained of left breast pain less than a month after her booster, which is being worked up.

Elderly Woman – Cough, Shortness of Breath, Emphysema

A thin and previously very active and healthy woman in her 90s received her shots in April and May. She said she has been sick ever since. She went seeking medical care in May for a new cough. In June, she had new shortness of breath. She began using inhalers. Workups for COVID were repeatedly negative, except she ended up with a new diagnosis of emphysema. Emphysema is typical for a 90-year-old, you say? I say not when she never smoked, and the sudden onset to life-changing severity was in one month. Emphysema and chronic obstructive bronchitis typically gradually worsen over several years or decades, not in a couple of weeks. That would be a very rare case.

Middle-Aged Man – Health Problems Ever Since

A man in his 50s has had many issues here in this book. He first had a severe case of shingles, followed by blood pressure elevation, then neck and shoulder pain, followed by back and leg pain. These issues required extra medical visits, new medications, and some referrals over the year following his shots. My guess is there are thousands, perhaps millions, just like him, with variations in their symptom timing.

Final Thoughts

I have several chronic patients with emphysema or pulmonary fibrosis or chronic obstructive lung disease who had recurrent or ongoing bronchitis for weeks to months after their shots. If they have some lung inflammation in their chronic disease and now they have more, they would have more trouble with flare-ups. Spike could cause high blood pressure in the lungs or pulmonary arterial hypertension (2). Interstitial lung disease has also been seen after these shots (3).

People tell you things when you're a nurse. I have had a dozen friends tell me they, their adult child, or extended family member has been having ongoing pain or health problems outside of work. All of these people received the shots. Interesting that none of my friends who did not receive the shots are having these new or worse health problems. I know four people outside of work and suspect another five who had a family member or extended family member pass shortly after their injections. I have also known five different people outside of work who have suffered a stroke in 2021, whereas in previous years, I personally knew of three over ten years. Each person believes they are the only ones who are experiencing devastating medical problems in themselves or their families, not realizing that millions, likely worldwide, are going through the same thing, in my opinion. I hear the repetitious stories day after day. We may never know this side of heaven, but who is investigating? Every news item or article in mainstream sources will always say if and when the person had a COVID illness, but if they did not have COVID, they would not say so, nor will they say when they had their shots. The escalation in nearly every illness seems to be blamed on 'long-haul' COVID. How convenient. The people in this book did not have COVID illness but had the shots. Also convenient to the mainstream narrative is counting vaccine deaths as COVID deaths (4).

Chapter 20
CHILDREN

Healthy Children

Healthy children have a two in a million, or one in 500,000, chance of dying of COVID (1). Healthy boys have a *1 in 2,563* chance of getting hospitalized for Myocarditis after these vaccines, which prompted a few countries to reduce vaccine requirements for the young (2). The rate of myocarditis is changing as time goes on, so the publication of this book is likely to be much higher because more children are being vaccinated, so we are slowly seeing a clearer picture. Other countries, such as Germany and Norway, do not recommend the vaccination of children due to the few clinical trials, early adverse events, and unknown long-term effects on boys (3). Some boys will never be the same (4), and some have died from this vaccine-induced myocarditis (2). There have been over 21,000 reports to VAERS for this one adverse related effect alone, with about 7,000 reports on people under the age of 43 and over 1,000 reports on ages 18 and under (5). As you read this book, keep in mind the number continues to grow. We will never know the actual number because historically and currently, VAERS and other health systems reporting are inadequate and severe under-reporting has been well established (6,7). There is extremely limited study of children on other possible adverse events.

Governmental Reporting

I can hear naysayers now. Again, they say VAERS is passive and can be totally coincidental. Why were there *exponentially* more reports than all other vaccines *combined* in the system's history? Indeed they aren't *all* coincidences. I say, then *where can* they be reported, taken seriously, and researched adequately? Why is there already so much research on heart conditions and so many lives lost at a young age in 2021? Watch out for escalation in childhood death in 2022-23 in countries that give these experimental gene therapy shots to children and toddlers. I agree VAERS is inadequate for capturing actual numbers, and even with low reporting numbers, the initial government studies of VAERS data are often found in error. For example, post COVID inoculation miscarriage rates were *7-8 times higher* than initial reports upon a closer review of the information (8). Some have already found data wiped from VAERS, that is now unsearchable but was previously easily found.

Our government inflated COVID illness, hospitalization, and death numbers, as is outlined by this Harvard research physician and study discussion (7). State and local governments are now reducing their total COVID death counts. One California *county* alone recently admitted they over-counted deaths by 400 people (9). Massachusetts reduced its COVID death number by 3,681 people (10). Massachusetts is a small state compared to California. If we estimate and extrapolate that over US states and territories, we have a *conservative reduction of nearly 200,000 deaths*. This counting trouble has occurred abroad, with the small United Kingdom counting deaths as COVID deaths regardless of how much time elapsed between illness and death. After catching this error, the UK reduced its death count by 5,000 (11).

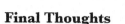

Final Thoughts

When did a generation request the sacrifice of their young for fear of the old? Even worse, if early treatment for COVID illness were given and broadly utilized, there would have been even fewer deaths. If the media and large corporations hadn't regurgitated it constantly, fear of this illness would be negligible, making the sacrifice of the young to this mass experiment a completely unnecessary tragedy (12). Sweden and Denmark offer this experimental gene therapy only to those 12 years old and up (13). The Hospital for Sick Children in Ontario has official guidance on post-shot heart risks and effects in children (14). Finally, if you decide to vaccinate your child or infant in the future, you are supposed to be given this FDA Fact Sheet to read first (15). Like all other vaccines and medications, you should be able to ask for the package insert, review it if you want to, and ask your provider questions. Your provider should not disrespect you for asking questions, get angry, mock you, or refuse to discuss your concerns. If they do, they either don't have the answers, don't know them, don't want to know and thus are inept at their job, or are coerced to follow the narrative. Of course there are some medical professionals who simply love their paycheck so will cower to big employers' mandates, sad to say. I hope some more of those providers, and some of the public, will respectfully but clearly write and meet with administrators, CEOs, CFOs, public health officials, and policy makers.

I carry one side of an old box of surgical masks in my purse sometimes and in my pocket other times. It states clearly on it that the masks do not prevent the spread of bacteria, viruses and infection. It is a box from early 2020. Now, many box manufacturers have removed this statement. The CDC studied 2 hairdressers who worked next to each other. A study from Europe was nearly 4,000 people. The CDC said masks work based on 2 hairstylists. I'm going with the 4,000 and the box that has read that masks don't prevent the spread of infection. Especially since the box has said this throughout my 30 year career, until 2021. I cannot complete this book without warning of the lasting damage to children and parents of young children wearing masks.

Facial skin staphylococcus infections, dental infections, recurring upper respiratory infections, overwhelming anxiety and depression, obsessive/compulsive disorders, and suicides have skyrocketed in children.. and adults. Many doctors made videos warning about the physical and psychological dangers and uselessness of masks to stop viruses and were canceled from all platforms. Journalists and television 'news' reporters are controlled by their employer who is controlled by their sponsors. You must realize that even your local medical school and your government has a sponsor in some form. Most professional medical organizations events and agendas are sponsored by pharmaceutical companies.

Viruses are so very microscopically tiny, so tiny they easily pass around and through a surgical or cloth mask...or two. You breathe in more moisture, mask particles, and carbon dioxide in a mask. Occupational Health and Safety Administration folks know that all masks had to be inspected for employees in years past, for safety related to all these issues. Suddenly, in 2020, OSHA folks were silent. Please, stop masking, unless, like Dr Fauci said on 60 Minutes in March 2020, it might make you feel better, but nobody should be wearing masks...or something very close to that. Look it up. Change your browser if you cannot seem to find it. Try Brave, Rumble, BrandNewTube, just to name a few.

But even if it makes you feel better to wear a mask, don't train your child to fear breathing air for the rest of their life or feed lifelong anxiety, depression, and OCD in their developing hearts and minds. Worse, don't feed their social and emotional and developmental disability. The standards of timely development in infants and toddlers were lowered very recently. This is why. I am not criticizing you if you masked your child. I am sure you followed whom you thought you could trust. I am begging you to not be offended, and to research farther and wider, critically think, definitely discern, and protect your child. Nothing more.

Chapter 21

HIGH-RISK ELDERS TREATED EARLY AT HOME FOR ILLNESS - FULLY RECOVERED

Early COVID Treatment Matters

COVID can and should be treated early. If it is such a terrible worry, why wait until you are exhausted, dehydrated, and not breathing well, with potential organ damage already, to *start* treatment? It can be tricky, requiring closer attention in some people, yes. Yes, it can be critical in a very few who have very high risks, recent immune insults, or predispositions to complications. But, very, very often, it can be successfully treated if *treated early and adequately*.

I have successfully treated people of various ages, ranging from their thirties to some in their seventies, eighties, and nineties. The oldest was in her late 90s and had dementia. I had a couple of women who sought me after recovering from a check-up and had no home treatment. Before they got sick, they were of a healthy weight and were active for their age and generally quite health conscious. I treated a few folks in their eighties and nineties with heart conditions. Several were in their seventies with heart conditions, diabetes, and lung conditions. I had folks in their fifties and sixties, many diabetic and/or obese with high blood pressure, high cholesterol, and various other health issues. I had one woman go to the hospital, but her husband told me she didn't take any of the medications or supplements and wasn't drinking fluids or walking intermittently, as was advised. He followed the home care instructions as was advised, and took the medication, and she didn't. She spent a few days hospitalized, but she was doing fine a couple weeks later at follow-up.

One spouse of a deceased man said that the TV news claimed there is no treatment for COVID except to go to the hospital so they went to the hospital and did not call me. I have also had a couple people tell me that their spouse, who was not a patient in my office, died of COVID in the hospital after no treatment was given by urgent care centers or their own doctor, despite their repeated asking for help. One unvaccinated, elderly, new patient died. He hadn't been to a doctor in decades, was morbidly obese, drank a lot of alcohol, and was an uncontrolled diabetic. The other couple of deaths were vaccinated, obese men in their 80s, beyond the average age of death in the US, who died in rehab or returned to the hospital from rehab. So their acute covid illness was behind them, but they remained weak and frail. Their cause of death would be labeled covid 19, even three or four months later. Now in the good old days, if someone fell and broke their hip, and died of pneumonia three months later because they were laid up since the fall, their primary cause of death would be pneumonia, not a hip fracture. See the difference in death counts, ..which began in March of 2020?

COVID Treatments Work

I treated most people with medications and/or supplements, depending on their age, risks, symptoms, and trajectory of the illness, quite specific home-care instructions and monitoring parameters, and extra calls or texts to check on them and guide them. A few needed oxygen for a few to several days. I referred over a dozen high-risk people to get monoclonal antibodies. However, I still treated them with medications while they waited for their appointment, especially since some of them were delayed or canceled for unknown reasons. Most of the people I treated with medications did not get monoclonal antibodies. Either there was no availability, or they just wanted to try the home management and medicine. Two men I had referred for monoclonal antibodies said they felt so good after taking the medications that they didn't think they needed to keep their appointments for monoclonal treatment. Because they were diabetic and one was morbidly obese, I talked them into keeping that appointment, and they fully recovered. All of my patients who took the medications *very early on* in the illness recovered quicker and had fewer lingering symptoms. Those who refused early medications typically had symptoms hang around much longer or claimed long haul Covid. I'll never forget one woman I knew who had recovered very slowly after hospitalization and commented to another woman who had been treated early at home. The first woman couldn't believe how quickly she recovered and was surprised to see her having a new urge to get healthy and lose weight, and going to the gym and working out shortly after her illness.

I individualized the AAPS protocol (Association of American Physicians and Surgeons, aapsonline.org) or the FLCCC protocol (Front Line COVID-19 Critical Care Alliance, COVID19criticalcare.com) for my patients. I added over the counter histamine blockers when needed according to the person's risks and symptom presentation. I am so grateful to the physicians who created these protocols and inspired other providers, such as myself, to treat people and prevent severe illnesses. Oh, the lives that could be less debilitated and the lives that could have been saved with early treatment, if only it weren't so hushed and controlled. These protocols include medication that some other countries have even adopted as first-line treatment (1). But see, if these protocols were widely known and used, there would be no emergency or need for rushed, experimental new inoculations.

How many of you know people, or perhaps you yourself, give your cat or dog medicines? I have a friend who gives her cat insulin injections three times a day, it is not a usual human dose of insulin! I have a friend who gives her dog heart medications, the same drugs people take, but it is not a human dose! Horses, of course, weigh more than humans, so their medicines are dosed much higher when weight based. Millions of Americans give their animals medicines daily- antibiotics, insulin, neuroleptics, antivirals, etc., etc.- but the medicine is weight based! Yet, our own government deceives, mocks, and repeats the narrative so much they actually convinced tens of millions. There has been over 70 studies in humans, showing that the 'horse medicine' was very effective to save lives, reduce hospitalizations, and reduce the duration and severity of the illness, when given in a human, weight based dose! Nevermind that this medicine has been given to humans billions of times before 2020 around the world and is one of the safest drugs of all time, is standard care in over a dozen countries with much lower death rates than ours, and the discoverer of this medicine won a Nobel peace prize. These studies and this information was canceled from 'mainstream' media and your 'news' feed.

I did know a couple of people and hear stories from friends about someone who had passed while hospitalized for COVID. They were not treated early at home. I heard of a local child who died from COVID. It was widely reported that she was a healthy, ordinary, young girl. She was not. She was very obese and looked at least ten years older than her age. This might come across as cold, but we must face many hard facts regardless of our perspective. We also need to discern and sometimes research hard, often repeated, and quick dismissals. We must investigate beyond the top hits and often beyond the first page of the old browsers. Obesity is a known killer, contributing to more than 350,000 deaths every year, year after year for over a decade before COVID even came along. Obesity alone nearly triples the chance of dying from COVID (2).

They were either sent home by urgent care clinics to 'push fluids', 'take Tylenol', and 'go to the hospital if you get short of breath' or were so unhealthy or obese beforehand that they were hospitalized within just a few days of getting symptoms. Obesity is one of the highest risks (3,5,6). The death rate of the hospitalized was nearly 18% (4,8). For that matter, the death rate in the US was very poor compared to many other countries (5,6,7). So, why the war on the freedom to prescribe and the freedom to share benefits and early evidence? People are dying from Covid, so they keep saying without evidence, two years later. Still, there are exceptionally few autopsies. But no, sir, there will be no treatment for Covid until you are ready to collapse. So, we learned nothing in two years? Seems there is a pattern of not learning anything new or helpful for many diseases lately. Or the strong powers that be ensure nothing will be learned? You decide.

I treated more unvaccinated 'Delta' cases than vaccinated, nearly 60% unvaccinated and 40% vaccinated. Regardless, they all needed almost the same treatment. For 'Omicron' cases, the vast majority were triple vaccinated and some quadruple vaccinated. Again, they all needed nearly the same treatment, with some variations in medication and follow-up attention depending on their condition and health risks. When this illness is actually treated early, using proven and often used protocols, preferably starting day 1-3, most people do well. Even most old people. Since most people recover well, especially with early treatment, it further emphasizes the severe health risks of either the shot's ingredients or the manufactured spike protein to the vessels, nerves, organs, body, and thus one's life, in my opinion.

Physicians and the Public Coerced

Physicians were coerced to assign COVID deaths, and autopsies were denied. I have had people tell me the health department coerced them, calling them repeatedly to get them to say their deceased loved one *might* have had a COVID symptom. It is now well known that COVID deaths were over-counted from day one, and many states have reduced their numbers of previously assigned COVID deaths. US deaths were counted differently than they have been counted for the nearly the last 20 years (9). Still, today, if you google this, you'll likely find nothing. There is much coercion at post shot death as well, because life insurance may not pay out in some cases if the cause is an experimental gene therapy. Finally, post COVID death certificates can garner extra family payouts, so incentivizing the labeling of death as COVID.

Final Thoughts

So here we have piles of peril close to mRNA acquired spike protein in those who did *not* have COVID illness. Please know that I listed only a handful of supportive studies to reference in each chapter. At least a thousand studies discuss potential perilous problems (10). More studies are coming out all the time. Will your evening news share that with you? Will our own governmental organizations? Will your doctor even hear about it? Has your provider asked you the dates of your shots before the onset of your new or much worsened health problems in 2021 or early 2022? Spike protein is spike protein. I don't care how a person gets it. It can be gasoline on your one flame of inflammation or the trigger on your immune system. Some very healthy may do well, as is survival of the fittest, but many have not and will not.

Peace to you and yours. Time will tell us all the Truth.

Resources and Support Sites

react19.org

This organization is doing research you can be involved in or read about, both post COVID illness or post-vaccination injury.

realnotrare.com

This organization offers much information and testimonies.

truthforhealth.org

This amazing organization offers vaccine injury reporting world-wide in English, Spanish and Chinese and other excellent supportive information on medical freedom and all things Covid.

c19vaxreactions.com

This organization was co-started by retired NFL player Ken Ruettgers after his wife and others were repeatedly ignored by pharmaceutical companies upon reporting their adverse reactions during the clinical trial stages.

NVICP National Vaccine Injury and Compensation Program

This government program has paid over 4 billion dollars to victims and their families of vaccine injury, disability, or death. This program was established in 1986 because litigation threatened pharmaceutical companies and created vaccine hesitancy (1). When enacted, it gave pharmaceutical companies complete immunity so no one could sue them for a vaccine injury. For every vaccine you take, 75 cents or more of the cost goes to this fund to pay others who have been harmed (1). So, you or your insurance company pay into the fund. Suppose childhood COVID vaccines are added to the pediatric schedule. In that case, the NVICP will be the only recourse for help as the pharmaceutical companies cannot be sued, despite these vaccines being new and experimental. The complete study trials of these new 'vaccines' were originally supposed to be completed in early 2023, which is still extremely rushed compared to the normal course of a vaccine development. If you weren't told that results would not be known until then, you didn't receive informed consent when you received yours.

VAERS Vaccine Adverse Event Reporting System

Medical providers are supposed to report suspected reactions on VAERS. How can they even begin to suspect if they don't ask for dates? How can they do this if they don't know about this site or the expectation to do so? What if the patient suspects but the doctor doesn't or refuses to consider it? What if the doctor refuses to discuss this with the patient? I have reported some of the people in this book and continue to do so slowly. It is very time-consuming and, of course, on my own time. Please report yourself or your loved one if the doctor won't acknowledge what you believe to be your highly likely or near certain injury from any COVID vaccine or other vaccine. Don't report that your arm where the needle went in has been slightly sore for two days. Do report lingering side effects, life-changing or recurring illness, debility, unexpected new diagnoses, emergency room visits, or frequent doctor visits shortly after shots. Talk to your doctor calmly and with some research if possible. Find another doctor if he curses you or refuses to discuss your health concern. Find out your lab results to report, if applicable. You will need the lot number and dates of the shots and have to clearly describe the dates of symptoms and health issues. You should get a confirmation from VAERS when you are done.

Recommendation

I suggest you also go to the other sites listed here and enter your testimony there. It has been challenging to learn quality data, duplicate a search, and retrieve previously entered persons on VAERS, making it suspect or inefficient, or inadequate for tracking and aggregating the reporting (2). Further, despite exponentially more reports to VAERS for these new types of 'vaccines' than all other previous vaccines in our lifetimes combined, and although VAERS is known to receive only a tiny fraction of actual cases, some of the powerful enigmas somehow don't see safety signals or trends. According to VAERS, there have been 1,249,929 total adverse reactions (3) and 23,753 deaths (4) associated with these new injections as of April 22, 2022. Remember, these are likely a roughly and repeatedly estimated 1-10% of reality because most people don't know to report here. Many doctors do not report, nor will they ever have time to. New vaccines were pulled off the market in prior years after just a few dozen reported injuries or deaths, but not in 2021. If you have never heard this, or much of what is discussed in this book, you must consider changing all your news sources. We must expand our sources of information, not tighten them. Consider independent news agencies, which are often harassed and vandalized. Consider independent researchers and physicians, who are not paid nor bribed by powerful enigmas and some of whom are risking their livelihoods and lives to investigate the science, share research, and treat people.

You will hear constant rebuttal to VAERS numbers. Some folks dismiss VAERS, year after year and constantly now, saying that anyone can report anything to VAERS, but that does not mean the vaccine caused their injury, new health problem, or death. Perhaps they never read the website itself, which says despite its flaws, VAERS is "very important in monitoring vaccine safety" (5). They might even say car accidents and possible stomach viruses or joint pains and chest pain are reported, and these obviously have nothing to do with the shots one receives because they happen every day. While the previous statement is true, those who constantly refute and dismiss VAERS seem to never concede that unless some of these things are aggregated, investigated, and researched, which is supposedly the purpose of VAERS, then there is no proof that the vaccine did not cause the reported health problem or death.

Further, if VAERS is so inept and a failure at tracking all these years and still today, what do they suggest for reporting possible, likely, and specific adverse effects, such as an entirely unexpected death within 24 hours? Or such as constant, piercing ringing in the ears followed by a deadly car accident within two to three weeks? Or trouble to stand and walking without getting dizzy and terrible joint pain that constantly keeps you on the couch? If autopsies aren't done, how do we know what caused their car accident? Are car accident rates up? Why are ER and urgent visits for chest pain, high blood pressure, various clots, and uncontrolled pain escalated? Are autoimmune illnesses or symptoms on an unusual rise? Cancer has certainly risen in my own experience. Finally, if VAERS is so inept and inaccurate, why wasn't a new and improved system implemented before the roll-out of brand new, experimental, gene-based inoculations? Yes, they are indeed gene-based (6), which is just another word that is quickly refuted or mocked, yet the truth. They are also still laden with risk, despite holding possible improvements for the future (6).

Compensation for Injury

Seeking compensation for vaccine injury? No one can guarantee you will be compensated, especially since these shots were given mass population permissions under emergency use and are not regularly FDA approved. You can start here: https://www.hrsa.gov/vaccine-compensation/index.html.

Resources for Finding Truth and Help:

- **truthforhealth.org**
- **Myfreedoctor.com**
- **flccc.net**
- **AAPSonline.org**
- **doctors4covidethics.org**
- **www.trialsitenews.com**
- **ipaknowledge.org**
- **Dr.Robert Malone**
- **Dr. Peter McCullough**
- **Dr. Stella Immanuel**
- **Dr. Sherry Tenpenny**
- **Dr. Ryan Cole**
- **Children's Health Defense**
- **Icandecide.org**
- **physiciansforinformedconsent.org**
- **Steve Kirsch**
- **Dr. David Martin**

There were over 17K doctors last year and more are coming along all the time, to the truth.

Final Thoughts

I realize some will defame me and say I'm peddling misinformation, but hey, we are all entitled to our opinion, aren't we? Let's talk about it. Let's continue the discussion without hiding. Let's listen. Accept debate when an esteemed physician asks you for it (7). Accept debate when Steve Kirsch asks you and will even pay you a million bucks for it! Maybe your misinformation is my information, and my information is your misinformation. It will stay that way forever with closed minds, cancellations, and calloused insults. Even if you dismiss me and all the resources in this chapter, the people in this book, and the backed-up medical system, what will you do with all your new health problems? With all your family's and friends' new health problems? With the unexpected early retirements and deaths? With medical discrimination? With the mysterious rise in all-cause mortality, even in the young, since 2021? The choice is yours. Just let others keep theirs. Understand a significant breach of medical ethics has taken place, doctors have been threatened, health care workers have been coerced and gagged, and effective treatments have been canceled (7).

Surely you know someone who was heavily coerced into taking the shots just to keep their job. I hear stories of discrimination and coercion regularly. Coercion is illegal, especially when it comes to experimental medical interventions. It is federal law:

21 U.S.C.§ S360bbb-3 (The FD&C Act), 21 C.F.R. § 50.20 21 C.F.R. § 50.23, 21 C.F.R. § 50.25, 21 C.F.R. 50.27, 18 U.S. Code Sect 2331 Sub 802

Coercion from corruption has flourished, thus lawlessness is prevailing and people are dying and are harmed.

Whatever you do, may you find the Way to healing and abundant Life.

Additional Resources

Kadwalwala M, Chadha B, Ortoleva J, Joyce M. Multimodality imaging and histopathology in a young man presenting with fulminant lymphocytic myocarditis and cardiogenic shock after mRNA-1273 vaccination. BMJ Case Rep. 2021 Nov 30;14(11):e246059. doi: 10.1136/bcr-2021-246059. PMID: 34848416; PMCID: PMC8634223.

Ismail II, Salama S. A systematic review of cases of CNS demyelination following COVID-19 vaccination. J Neuroimmunol. 2022 Jan 15;362:577765. doi: 10.1016/j.jneuroim.2021.577765. Epub 2021 Nov 9. PMID: 34839149; PMCID: PMC8577051.

David M. Smadja, Qun-Ying Yue, Richard Chocron, Olivier Sanchez, Agnes Lillo-Le Louet, Vaccination against COVID-19: insight from arterial and venous thrombosis occurrence using data from VigiBase

European Respiratory Journal 2021 58: 2100956; DOI: 10.1183/13993003.00956-2021

Luigi Cari, Mahdieh Naghavi Alhosseini, Paolo Fiore, Sabata Pierno, Sabrina Pacor, Alberta Bergamo, Gianni Sava, Giuseppe Nocentini, Cardiovascular, neurological, and pulmonary events following vaccination with the BNT162b2, ChAdOx1 nCoV-19, and Ad26.COV2.S vaccines: An analysis of European data, Journal of Autoimmunity, Volume 125,2021,102742, ISSN 0896-8411,https://doi.org/10.1016/j.jaut.2021.102742.

Fatma Elrashdy, Murtaza M. Tambuwala, Sk. Sarif Hassan, Parise Adadi, Murat Seyran, Tarek Mohamed Abd El-Aziz, Nima Rezaei, Amos Lal, Alaa A.A. Aljabali, Ramesh Kandimalla, Nicolas G. Bazan, Gajendra Kumar Azad, Samendra P. Sherchan, Pabitra Pal Choudhury, Ángel Serrano-Aroca, Kazuo Takayama, Gaurav Chauhan, Damiano Pizzol, Debmalya Barh, Pritam Kumar Panda, Yogendra K. Mishra, Giorgio Palù, Kenneth Lundstrom, Elrashdy M. Redwan, Vladimir N. Uversky, Autoimmunity roots of the thrombotic events after COVID-19 vaccination, Autoimmunity Reviews, Volume 20, Issue 11, 2021, 102941, ISSN 1568-9972, https://doi.org/10.1016/j.autrev.2021.102941.

Higgins-Dunn N. FDA staff recommends watching for Bell's palsy in Moderna and Pfizer vaccine recipients. CNBC Dec. 15, 2020.

CDC. Allergic Reactions Inducing Anaphylaxis After Receipt of the First Dose of Pfizer-BioNTech COVID-9 Vaccine – United States, December 14-23, 2020. MMWR Jan. 15, 2021; 70(2): 46-51.

Rutkowski K, Mirakian R et al. Adverse reactions to COVID-19 vaccines: a practical approach. Clin Exp Allergy 2021; 51(6): 770-777.

Kania K, Ambrosius W, Kupczyk ET, Kozubski W. Acute disseminated encephalomyelitis in a patient vaccinated against SARS-CoV-2. Annals of Clinical and Translational Neurology Sept. 4, 2021.

Bussel JB, Connors JM, Cines DB et al. Thrombosis with Thrombo-cytopenia Syndrome (also termed Vaccine-induced Thrombotic Thrombocytopenia). American Society of Hematology Aug. 12, 2021.

Classen JB. US COVID-19 Vaccines Proven to Cause More Harm than Good Based on Pivotal Clinical Trial Data Analyzed Using the Proper Scientific Endpoint, "All Cause Severe Morbidity." Trend Int Med 2021; 1(1): 1-6.

Fisher BL. Healthy Mom, 39, in Utah Dies of Organ Failure Four Days After Moderna COVID Vaccination. The Vaccine Reaction Mar. 15, 2021.

Fisher BL. More Deaths Reported to VAERS Following COVID-19 Vaccinations Than for Any Other Vaccine. The Vaccine Reaction July 11, 2021. 24 Menon P. New Zealand reports first death linked to Pfizer/BioNTech COVID-19

García-Azorín D, Do TP, Gantenbein AR, Hansen JM, Souza MNP, Obermann M, Pohl H, Schankin CJ, Schytz HW, Sinclair A, Schoonman GG, Kristoffersen ES. Delayed headache after COVID-19 vaccination: a red flag for vaccine induced cerebral venous thrombosis. J Headache Pain. 2021 Sep 17;22(1):108. doi: 10.1186/s10194-021-01324-5. PMID: 34535076; PMCID: PMC8446734. (Onset HA 7-9.7 days)

Bleier BS, Ramanathan M, Lane AP. COVID-19 Vaccines May Not Prevent Nasal SARS-CoV-2 Infection and Asymptomatic Transmission. Otolaryngology–Head and Neck Surgery. 2021;164(2):305-307. doi:10.1177/0194599820982633

Bibliography

Introduction

1 Kowarz E, Krutzke L, Reis J, et al. "Vaccine-Induced COVID-19 Mimicry" Syndrome: Splice reactions within the SARS-CoV-2 Spike open reading frame result in Spike protein variants that may cause thromboembolic events in patients immunized with vector-based vaccines. Research Square; 2021. DOI: 10.21203/rs.3.rs-558954/v1.

2 De Michele M, Kahan J, Berto I, Schiavo OG, Iacobucci M, Toni D, Merkler AE. Cerebrovascular Complications of COVID-19 and COVID-19 Vaccination. Circ Res. 2022 Apr 15;130(8):1187-1203. doi: 10.1161/CIRCRESA-HA.122.319954. Epub 2022 Apr 14. PMID: 35420916; PMCID: PMC9005103.

3 Liu, J., Wang, J., Xu, J. et al. Comprehensive investigations revealed consistent pathophysiological alterations after vaccination with COVID-19 vaccines. Cell Discov 7, 99 (2021). https://doi.org/10.1038/s41421-021-00329-3

4 https://doi.org/10.1136/bmj-2021-068414 -links to study delay of presentation of symptoms

5 Abstract 10712: Observational Findings of PULS Cardiac Test Findings for Inflammatory Markers in Patients Receiving mRNA Vaccines | Circulation (ahajournals.org)

6
https://www.ahrq.gov/research/findings/factsheets/primary/pcwork3/index.html

7 Indiana life insurance CEO says deaths are up 40% among people ages 18-64 | Indiana | thecentersquare.com

8 https://www.kusi.com/there-was-an-unexpected-40-increase-in-all-cause-deaths-in-2021

9 COVID-19 Yellow Card Data | UKColumn

10 Vaccination consequences: Health insurance BKK writes letter to Paul-Ehrlich-Institut (berliner-zeitung.de)

11 Vaccines and Related Biological Products Advisory Committee October 22, 2020 Meeting Presentation- COVID19 CBER Plans for Monitoring Vaccine Safety and Effectiveness (fda.gov) https://www.fda.gov/media/143557/download

Chapter 1

1 E.E. Walsh, R.W. Frenck Jr., A.R. Falsey, N. Kitchin, J. Absalon, A. Gurtman, S. Lockhart, K. Neuzil, M.J. Mulligan, R. Bailey, K.A. Swanson, P. Li, K. Koury, W. Kalina, D. Cooper, C. Fontes-Garfias, P.Y. Shi, Ö. Türeci, K.R. Tompkins, K.E. Lyke, V. Raabe, P.R. Dormitzer, K.U. Jansen, U. Şahin, W.C. Gruber. Safety and immunogenicity of two RNA-Based COVID-19 vaccine candidates N. Engl. J. Med., 383 (2020), pp. 2439-2450

2 COVID-19 vaccines induce severe hemolysis in paroxysmal nocturnal hemoglobinuria: https://ashpublications.org/blood/article/137/26/3670/475905/COVID-19-vaccines-induce-severe-hemolysis-in

3 Collection of complement-mediated and autoimmune-mediated hematologic conditions after SARS-CoV-2 vaccination: https://ashpublications.org/bloodadvances/article/5/13/2794/476324/Autoimmune-and-complement-mediated-hematologic

Fedorowski A: Postural orthostatic tachycardia syndrome: clinical presentation, aetiology and management. J Intern Med. 2019, 285:352-66. 10.1111/joim.12852

4 Reddy S, Reddy S, Arora M (May 04, 2021) A Case of Postural Orthostatic Tachycardia Syndrome Secondary to the Messenger RNA COVID-19 Vaccine. Cureus 13(5): e14837. doi:10.7759/cureus.14837

5 Brinth L, Theibel AC, Pors K, Mehlsen J: Suspected side effects to the quadrivalent human papilloma vaccine. Danish Med J. 2015, 62:5064.

6 Blitshteyn S: Postural tachycardia syndrome following human papillomavirus vaccination. Eur J Neurol. 2014, 21:135-9. 10.1111/ene.12272

7 Neurological side effects of SARS-CoV-2 vaccinations - Finsterer - 2022 - Acta Neurologica Scandinavica - https://doi.org/10.1111/ane.13550

8 Aphasia seven days after second dose of an mRNA-based SARS-CoV-2 vaccine - PubMed (nih.gov) https://doi.org/10.1016/j.hest.2021.06.001

9 Wiley Online Library SARS-CoV-2 vaccines are not free of neurological side effects - Finsterer - 2021 - Acta Neurologica Scandinavica - Wiley Online Library https://doi.org/10.1111/ane.13451

10 Bussel JB, Connors JM, Cines DB et al. Thrombosis with Thrombocytopenia Syndrome (also termed Vaccine-induced Thrombotic Thrombocytopenia). American Society of Hematology Aug. 12, 2021.

11 Dr. Sucharit Bhakdi Interview - COVID Vaccine Blood Clot Risk Was Known, Ignored & Buried (thelastamericanvagabond.com)

12 Acute Myocardial Injury Following COVID-19 Vaccination: A Case Report and Review of Current Evidence from Vaccine Adverse Events Reporting System Database - Anasua Deb, John Abdelmalek, Kenneth Iwuji, Kenneth Nugent, 2021 (sagepub.com) https://doi.org/10.1177% 2F215013272110 29230

13 Troponin https://www.ncbi.nlm.nih.gov/books/NBK507805/

14 BMJ 2021; 373:n958 Thrombosis after COVID-19 vaccination BMJ 2021; 373 doi: https://doi.org/10.1136/bmj.n958 (Published 14 April 2021)

15 Brandon Goodwin: 1000% the COV Vax Caused His Blood Clots, NBA Told Him to Keep Quiet! (independentsentinel.com)

16 https://www.docdroid.net/xq0Z8B0/pfizer-report-japanese-government-pdf

17 https://www.regulations.gov/document/FDA-2020-N-1898-0246 Dr Whalen

18 https://www.youtube.com/watch?v=QZyBUmuIQP4 Dr Been Medical Lectures

19 Bikdeli B, Jiménez D, Demelo-Rodriguez P, Galeano-Valle F, Porras JA, Barba R, Ay C, Malý R, Braester A, Imbalzano E, Rosa V, Lecumberri R, Siniscalchi C, Fidalgo Á, Ortiz S, Monreal M, For The Riete Investigators. Venous Thrombosis within 30 Days after Vaccination against SARS-CoV-2 in a Multinational Venous Thromboembolism Registry. Viruses. 2022 Jan 18;14(2):178. doi: 10.3390/v14020178. PMID: 35215771; PMCID: PMC8878689.

20 https://investors.pfizer.com/Investors/Financials/Quarterly-Results/
s28.q4cdn.com

21 https://www.statista.com/statistics/314585/leading-pharmaceutical-products-
by-revenue-in-the-us/

22 Diogo Goulart Corrêa, Luis Alcides Quevedo Cañete, Gutemberg Augusto
Cruz dos Santos, Romulo Varella de Oliveira, Carlos Otávio Brandão, Luiz Celso
Hygino da Cruz. Neurological symptoms and neuroimaging alterations related with
COVID-19 vaccine: Cause or coincidence?,Clinical Imaging,Volume 80,2021,
348-352, ISSN 0899-7071, https://doi.org/10.1016/j.clinimag.2021.08.021.

Chapter 2

1 Jesse Santiano M.D.Don't Get Sick!Higher blood pressure after COVID shots
and why it happens (drjessesantiano.com)

2 Zappa M, Verdecchia P, Spanevello A, Visca D, Angeli F. Blood pressure increase
after Pfizer/BioNTech SARS-CoV-2 vaccine. Eur J Intern Med. 2021;90:111-113.
doi:10.1016/j.ejim.2021.06.013

3 Jeet Kaur R, Dutta S, Charan J, et al. Cardiovascular Adverse Events Reported
from COVID-19 Vaccines: A Study Based on WHO Database. Int J Gen Med.
2021;14:3909-3927. Published 2021 July 27. doi:10.2147/IJGM.S324349

4 Meylan S, Livio F, Foerster M, Genoud PJ, Marguet F, Wuerzner G; CHUV
COVID Vaccination Center. Stage III Hypertension in Patients After mRNA-
Based SARS-CoV-2 vaccination. Hypertension. 2021 Jun;77(6):e56-e57. Doi:
10.1161/HYPERTENSIONAHA.121.17316. Epub 2021 March 25. PMID:
33764160; PMCID: PMC8115421.

5 Suzuki YJ, Gychka SG. SARS-CoV-2 Spike Protein Elicits Cell Signaling in
Human Host Cells: Implications for Possible Consequences of COVID-19
Vaccines. Vaccines (Basel). 2021;9(1):36. Published 2021 January 11.
doi:10.3390/vaccines9010036

Chapter 3

1 Vaccines and Related Biological Products Advisory Committee October 22, 2020 Meeting Presentation- COVID19 CBER Plans for Monitoring Vaccine Safety and Effectiveness (fda.gov) https://www.fda.gov/media/143557/download

2 https://doi.org/10.1016/j.jpeds.2021.07.057

3 https://www.cdc.gov/coronavirus/2019-ncov/vaccines/safety/myocarditis.html

4 Mateusz Tajstra, Jerzy Jaroszewicz, Mariusz Gąsior, Acute Coronary Tree Thrombosis After Vaccination for COVID-19, JACC: Cardiovascular Interventions, Volume 14, Issue 9, 2021, Pages e103-e104, ISSN 1936-8798, https://doi.org/10.1016/j.jcin.2021.03.003

5 Talal Almas, Sarah Rehman, Eyad Mansour, Tarek Khedro, Ali Alansari, Jahanzeb Malik, Norah Alshareef, Vikneswaran Raj Nagarajan, Abdulla Hussain Al-Awaid, Reema Alsufyani, Majid Alsufyani, Ali Rifai, Ahlam Alzahrani, Dhineswaran Raj Nagarajan, Tala Abdullatif, Varman Gunasaegaram, Enaam Alzadjali, Arthi Subramanian, Abida Rahman, Yasar Sattar, Jason Galo, Hafeez Ul Hassan Virk, M. Chadi Alraies, Epidemiology, clinical ramifications, and cellular pathogenesis of COVID-19 mRNA-vaccination-induced adverse cardiovascular outcomes: A state-of-the-heart review, Biomedicine & Pharmacotherapy, Volume 149, 2022, 112843, ISSN 0753-3322, https://doi.org/10.1016/j.biopha.2022.112843.

6 Chamling, B., Vehof, V., Drakos, S. et al. Occurrence of acute infarct-like myocarditis following COVID-19 vaccination: just an accidental co-incidence or rather vaccination-associated autoimmune myocarditis?. Clin Res Cardiol 110, 1850–1854 (2021). https://doi.org/10.1007/s00392-021-01916-w

Chapter 4

1 Bari, Razmin, Bepari, Asim Kumar and Reza, Hasan Mahmud. "COVID-19: Lessons from Norway tragedy must be considered in vaccine rollout planning in least developed/developing countries" Open Medicine, vol. 16, no. 1, 2021, pp. 1168-1169. https://doi.org/10.1515/med-2021-0334

2 Khayat-Khoei, M., Bhattacharyya, S., Katz, J. et al. COVID-19 mRNA vaccination leading to CNS inflammation: a case series. J Neurol 269, 1093–1106 (2022). https://doi.org/10.1007/s00415-021-10780-7

3 Baldelli L, Amore G, Montini A, Panzera I, Rossi S, Cortelli P, Guarino M, Rinaldi R, D'Angelo R. Hyperacute reversible encephalopathy related to cytokine storm following COVID-19 vaccine. J Neuroimmunol. 2021 Sep 15;358:577661. doi: 10.1016/j.jneuroim.2021.577661. Epub 2021 Jul 13. PMID: 34284342; PMCID: PMC8275470.

4 Abdulrahman F. Al-Mashdali, Yaser M. Ata, Nagham Sadik, Post-COVID-19 vaccine acute hyperactive encephalopathy with dramatic response to methylprednisolone: A case report, Annals of Medicine and Surgery, Volume 69, 2021, 102803, ISSN 2049-0801, https://doi.org/10.1016/j.amsu.2021.102803.

5 Zlotnik Yair, Gadoth Avi, Abu-Salameh Ibrahim, Horev Anat, Novoa Rosa, Ifergane Gal Case Report: Anti-LGI1 Encephalitis Following COVID-19 Vaccination Frontiers in Immunology VOLUME12 2022 https://www.frontiersin.org/articles/10.3389/fimmu.2021.813487,ISSN=1664-3224 DOI10.3389/fimmu.2021.813487

Chapter 5

1 Post COVID-19 vaccine small fiber neuropathy - Waheed - 2021 - Muscle & Nerve - Wiley Online Library https://doi.org/10.1002/mus.27251

Chapter 6

1 Tahir N, Koorapati G, Prasad S, Jeelani HM, Sherchan R, Shrestha J, Shayuk M. SARS-CoV-2 Vaccination-Induced Transverse Myelitis. Cureus. 2021 Jul 25;13(7):e16624. doi: 10.7759/cureus.16624. PMID: 34458035; PMCID: PMC8384391.

2 Vaccines and Related Biological Products Advisory Committee October 22, 2020 Meeting Presentation- COVID19 CBER Plans for Monitoring Vaccine Safety and Effectiveness (fda.gov) https://www.fda.gov/media/143557/download

3 Khan E, Shrestha AK, Colantonio MA, Liberio RN, Sriwastava S. Acute transverse myelitis following SARS-CoV-2 vaccination: a case report and review of literature. J Neurol. 2022 Mar;269(3):1121-1132. doi: 10.1007/s00415-021-10785-2. Epub 2021 Sep 5. PMID: 34482455; PMCID: PMC8418691.

4 Maniscalco GT, Manzo V, Di Battista ME, Salvatore S, Moreggia O, Scavone C, Capuano A. Severe Multiple Sclerosis Relapse After COVID-19 Vaccination: A Case Report. Front Neurol. 2021 Aug 10;12:721502. doi: 10.3389/fneur.2021.721502. PMID: 34447349; PMCID: PMC8382847.

5 Masoud Etemadifar, Amirhossein Akhavan Sigari, Nahad Sedaghat, Mehri Salari & Hosein Nouri (2021) Acute relapse and poor immunization following COVID-19 vaccination in a rituximab-treated multiple sclerosis patient, Human Vaccines & Immunotherapeutics, 17:10, 3481-3483, DOI: 10.1080/21645515.2021.1928463

Chapter 8

1 Román GC, Gracia F, Torres A, Palacios A, Gracia K, Harris D. Acute Transverse Myelitis (ATM):Clinical Review of 43 Patients With COVID-19-Associated ATM and 3 Post-Vaccination ATM Serious Adverse Events With the ChAdOx1 nCoV-19 Vaccine (AZD1222). Front Immunol. 2021 Apr 26;12:653786. doi: 10.3389/fimmu.2021.653786. PMID: 33981305; PMCID: PMC8107358.

2 Vaccines and Related Biological Products Advisory Committee October 22, 2020 Meeting Presentation- COVID19 CBER Plans for Monitoring Vaccine Safety and Effectiveness (fda.gov) https://www.fda.gov/media/143557/download

Chapter 9

1 Aldén M, Olofsson Falla F, Yang D, Barghouth M, Luan C, Rasmussen M, De Marinis Y. Intracellular Reverse Transcription of Pfizer BioNTech COVID-19 mRNA Vaccine BNT162b2 In Vitro in Human Liver Cell Line. *Current Issues in Molecular Biology.* 2022; 44(3):1115-1126. https://doi.org/10.3390/cimb44030073

2 Pomara C, Sessa F, Ciaccio M, Dieli F, Esposito M, Garozzo SF, Giarratano A, Prati D, Rappa F, Salerno M, Tripodo C, Zamboni P, Mannucci PM. Post-mortem findings in vaccine-induced thrombotic thombocytopenia. Haematologica 2021;106(8):2291-2293; https://doi.org/10.3324/haematol.2021.279075

3 Mateo Porres-Aguilar, Alejandro Lazo-Langner, Arturo Panduro, Misael Uribe, COVID-19 vaccine-induced immune thrombotic thrombocytopenia: An emerging cause of splanchnic vein thrombosis, Annals of Hepatology, Volume 23, 2021, 100356,ISSN 1665-2681, https://doi.org/10.1016/j.aohep.2021.100356.

4 Vuille-Lessard É, Montani M, Bosch J, Semmo N. Autoimmune hepatitis triggered by SARS-CoV-2 vaccination. J Autoimmun. 2021 Sep;123:102710. doi: 10.1016/j.jaut.2021.102710. Epub 2021 Jul 28. PMID: 34332438; PMCID: PMC8316013.

5 Ghielmetti M, Schaufelberger HD, Mieli-Vergani G, Cerny A, Dayer E, Vergani D, Terziroli Beretta-Piccoli B. Acute autoimmune-like hepatitis with atypical antimitochondrial antibody after mRNA COVID-19 vaccination: A novel clinical entity? J Autoimmun. 2021 Sep;123:102706. doi: 10.1016/j.jaut.2021.102706. Epub 2021 Jul 15. PMID: 34293683; PMCID: PMC8279947.

6 Garrido I, Lopes S, Simões MS, Liberal R, Lopes J, Carneiro F, Macedo G. Autoimmune hepatitis after COVID-19 vaccine - more than a coincidence. J Autoimmun. 2021 Dec;125:102741. doi: 10.1016/j.jaut.2021.102741. Epub 2021 Oct 26. PMID: 34717185; PMCID: PMC8547941.

7 Gloria Shwe Zin Tun, Dermot Gleeson, Amer Al-Joudeh, Asha Dube, Immune-mediated hepatitis with the Moderna vaccine, no longer a coincidence but confirmed, Journal of Hepatology, Volume 76, Issue 3, 2022, Pages 747-749, ISSN 0168-8278, https://doi.org/10.1016/j.jhep.2021.09.031.

8 Trogstad L, Robertson AH, Mjaaland S, Magnus P. Association between ChAdOx1 nCoV-19 vaccination and bleeding episodes: Large population-based cohort study. Vaccine. 2021 Sep 24;39(40):5854-5857. doi: 10.1016/j.vaccine.2021.08.055. Epub 2021 Aug 31. PMID: 34479760; PMCID: PMC8406020.

9 Rahim SEG, Lin JT, Wang JC. A case of gross hematuria and IgA nephropathy flare-up following SARS-CoV-2 vaccination. Kidney Int. 2021 Jul;100(1):238. doi: 10.1016/j.kint.2021.04.024. Epub 2021 Apr 28. PMID: 33932458; PMCID: PMC8079938.

10 Perrin P, Bassand X, Benotmane I, Bouvier N. Gross hematuria following SARS-CoV-2 vaccination in patients with IgA nephropathy. Kidney Int. 2021 Aug;100(2):466-468. doi: 10.1016/j.kint.2021.05.022. Epub 2021 Jun 1. PMID: 34087252; PMCID: PMC8166778.

11 Plasse R, Nee R, Gao S, Olson S. Acute kidney injury with gross hematuria and IgA nephropathy after COVID-19 vaccination. Kidney Int. 2021 Oct;100(4):944-945. doi: 10.1016/j.kint.2021.07.020. Epub 2021 Aug 3. PMID: 34352309; PMCID: PMC8329426.

Chapter 10

1 Does poor glycaemic control affect the immunogenicity of the COVID-19 vaccination in patients with type 2 diabetes: The CAVEAT study - Marfella - 2022 - Diabetes, Obesity and Metabolism - Wiley Online Library https://doi.org/10.1111/dom.14547

2 Liu, J., Wang, J., Xu, J. et al. Comprehensive investigations revealed consistent pathophysiological alterations after vaccination with COVID-19 vaccines. Cell Discov 7, 99 (2021). https://doi.org/10.1038/s41421-021-00329-3

3 Joob B, Wiwanitkit V. Change of blood viscosity after COVID-19 vaccination: estimation for persons with underlying metabolic syndrome. Int J Physiol Pathophysiol Pharmacol. 2021 Oct 15;13(5):148-151. PMID: 34868465; PMCID: PMC8611240.

Chapter 11

1 https://www.thegms.co/medical-ethics/medethics-rw-22021403.pdf

Chapter 12

1 Faissner, S., Richter, D., Ceylan, U. et al. COVID-19 mRNA vaccine induced rhabdomyolysis and fasciitis. J Neurol 269, 1774–1775 (2022). https://doi.org/10.1007/s00415-021-10768-3

2 Mahmoud Nassar, Howard Chung, Yarl Dhayaparan, Andrew Nyein, Bryan Jose Acevedo, Celestin Chicos, David Zheng, Mathieu Barras, Mahmoud Mohamed, Mostafa Alfishawy, Nso Nso, Vincent Rizzo, Eben Kimball, COVID-19 vaccine induced rhabdomyolysis: Case report with literature review,Diabetes & Metabolic Syndrome: Clinical Research & Reviews, Volume 15, Issue 4, 2021, 102170, ISSN 1871-4021, https://doi.org/10.1016/j.dsx.2021.06.007.

3 Hyun H, Song JY, Seong H, Yoon JG, Noh JY, Cheong HJ, Kim WJ. Polyarthralgia and Myalgia Syndrome after ChAdOx1 nCOV-19 Vaccination. J Korean Med Sci. 2021 Aug 30;36(34):e245. doi: 10.3346/jkms.2021.36.e245. PMID: 34463066; PMCID: PMC8405407.

Chapter 13

1 Acute abducens nerve palsy after COVID-19 vaccination: https://pubmed.ncbi.nlm.nih.gov/34044114/.

2 Transient oculomotor paralysis after administration of RNA-1273 messenger
vaccine for SARS-CoV-2 diplopia after COVID-19
vaccine: https://pubmed.ncbi.nlm.nih.gov/34369471/

3 Bell's palsy after Ad26.COV2.S COVID-19 vaccination: https://pubmed.ncbi.nlm.nih.gov/34014316/

4 Bell's palsy after COVID-19 vaccination: case
report: https://pubmed.ncbi.nlm.nih.gov/34330676/

5 A case of acute demyelinating polyradiculoneuropathy with bilateral facial palsy
following ChAdOx1 nCoV-19
vaccination: https://pubmed.ncbi.nlm.nih.gov/34272622/

6 Burrows A, Bartholomew T, Rudd J, Walker D. Sequential contralateral facial
nerve palsies following COVID-19 vaccination first and second doses. BMJ Case
Rep. 2021 Jul 19;14(7):e243829. doi: 10.1136/bcr-2021-243829. PMID: 34281950;
PMCID: PMC8291314.

Chapter 14

1 https://rarediseases.org/rare-diseases/henoch-schonlein-purpura/

2 Laure Badier, Albanie Toledano, Tiphaine Porel, Sylvain Dumond, Julien
Jouglen, Laurent Sailler, Haleh Bagheri, Guillaume Moulis, Margaux Lafaurie, IgA
vasculitis in adult patient following vaccination by ChadOx1 nCoV-19, Autoimmunity Reviews, Volume 20, Issue 11, 2021, 102951, ISSN 1568-9972,
https://doi.org/10.1016/j.autrev.2021.102951.

3 Erler, A., Fiedler, J., Koch, A., Heldmann, F. and Schütz, A. (2021), Leukocyto-
clastic Vasculitis After Vaccination With a SARS-CoV-2 Vaccine. Arthritis
Rheumatol, 73: 2188-2188. https://doi.org/10.1002/art.41910

4 Annabi, E., Dupin, N., Sohier, P., Garel, B., Franck, N., Aractingi, S., Guégan, S. and Oulès, B. (2021), Rare cutaneous adverse effects of COVID-19 vaccines: a case series and review of the literature. J Eur Acad Dermatol Venereol, 35: e847-e850. https://doi.org/10.1111/jdv.17578

5 Petechial rash associated with CoronaVac vaccination: first report of cutaneous side effects before phase 3 results: https://ejhp.bmj.com/content/early/2021/05/23/ejhpharm-2021-002794

6 Poulas K, Farsalinos K. Response to McMahon et al's "Cutaneous reactions reported after Moderna and Pfizer COVID-19 vaccination: A registry-based study of four hundred fourteen cases". J Am Acad Dermatol. 2022 Apr;86(4):e163-e164. doi: 10.1016/j.jaad.2021.09.071. Epub 2021 Nov 18. PMID: 34801633; PMCID: PMC8600750.

7 Desai HD, Sharma K, Shah A, Patoliya J, Patil A, Hooshanginezhad Z, Grabbe S, Goldust M. Can SARS-CoV-2 vaccine increase the risk of reactivation of Varicella zoster? A systematic review. J Cosmet Dermatol. 2021 Nov;20(11):3350-3361. doi: 10.1111/jocd.14521. PMID: 34719084; PMCID: PMC8597588.

8 Iwanaga J, Fukuoka H, Fukuoka N, Yutori H, Ibaragi S, Tubbs RS. A narrative review and clinical anatomy of herpes zoster infection following COVID-19 vaccination. Clin Anat. 2022 Jan;35(1):45-51. doi: 10.1002/ca.23790. Epub 2021 Oct 1. PMID: 34554601; PMCID: PMC8652627.

Chapter 15

1 Nicholas Fowler, Noe R. Mendez Martinez, Bernardo Velazquez Pallares, Ramiro S. Maldonado,Acute-onset central serous retinopathy after immunization with COVID-19 mRNA vaccine, American Journal of Ophthalmology Case Reports, Volume 23, 2021, 101136, ISSN 2451-9936, https://doi.org/10.1016/j.ajoc.2021.101136.

2 Pappaterra MC, Rivera EJ, Oliver AL. Transient Oculomotor Palsy Following the Administration of the Messenger RNA-1273 Vaccine for SARS-CoV-2 Diplopia Following the COVID-19 Vaccine. J Neuroophthalmol. 2021 Aug 4. doi: 10.1097/WNO.0000000000001369. Epub ahead of print. PMID:34369471.

3 De Michele M, Kahan J, Berto I, Schiavo OG, Iacobucci M, Toni D, Merkler AE. Cerebrovascular Complications of COVID-19 and COVID-19 Vaccination. Circ Res. 2022 Apr 15;130(8):1187-1203. doi: 10.1161/CIRCRESA-HA.122.319954. Epub 2022 Apr 14. PMID: 35420916; PMCID: PMC9005103.

Chapter 16

1 Management of Unilateral Axillary Lymphadenopathy Detected on Breast MRI in the Era of COVID-19 Vaccination - PubMed (nih.gov)
DOI: 10.2214/AJR.21.25604

2 https://www.audacy.com/podcasts/american-conservative-university-25894/dr-ryan-cole-alarming-cancer-trend-suggests-COVID-19-vaccines-alter-natural-immune-response-1231350527

3 https://rumble.com/vt62y6-COVID-19-a-second-opinion.html

4 Faermann R, Nissan N, Halshtok-Neiman O, Shalmon A, Gotlieb M, Yagil Y, Samoocha D, Friedman E, Sklair-Levy M. COVID-19 Vaccination Induced Lymphadenopathy in a Specialized Breast Imaging Clinic in Israel: Analysis of 163 cases. Acad Radiol. 2021 Sep;28(9):1191-1197. doi: 10.1016/j.acra.2021.06.003. Epub 2021 Jun 10. PMID: 34257025; PMCID: PMC8189756.

5 Mitchell OR, Couzins M, Dave R, Bekker J, Brennan PA. COVID-19 vaccination and low cervical lymphadenopathy in the two week neck lump clinic - a follow up audit. Br J Oral Maxillofac Surg. 2021 Jul;59(6):720-721. doi: 10.1016/j.b-joms.2021.04.008. Epub 2021 Apr 21. PMID: 33947605; PMCID: PMC8057932.

6 Abou-Foul AK, Ross E, Abou-Foul M, George AP. Cervical lymphadenopathy following coronavirus disease 2019 vaccine: clinical characteristics and implications for head and neck cancer services. J Laryngol Otol. 2021 Nov; 135 (11): 1025-1030. doi: 10.1017/S0022215121002462. Epub 2021 Sep 16. PMID: 34526175; PMCID: PMC8476898.

7 Placke JM, Reis H, Hadaschik E, Roesch A, Schadendorf D, Stoffels I, Klode J. Coronavirus disease 2019 vaccine mimics lymph node metastases in patients undergoing skin cancer follow-up: A monocentre study. Eur J Cancer. 2021 Sep;154:167-174. doi: 10.1016/j.ejca.2021.06.023. Epub 2021 Jun 26. PMID: 34280870; PMCID: PMC8233908.

8 Jiang H, Mei YF. SARS-CoV-2 Spike Impairs DNA Damage Repair and Inhibits V(D)J Recombination In Vitro. Viruses. 2021 Oct 13;13(10):2056. doi: 10.3390/v13102056. PMID: 34696485; PMCID: PMC8538446.

9 Singh N, Bharara Singh A. S2 subunit of SARS-nCoV-2 interacts with tumor suppressor protein p53 and BRCA: an in silico study. Transl Oncol. 2020;13(10):100814. doi:10.1016/j.tranon.2020.100814

10 Ye, Z., Shi, Y., Lees-Miller, S. P., & Tainer, J. A. (2021). Function and Molecular Mechanism of the DNA Damage Response in Immunity and Cancer Immunotherapy. Frontiers in immunology, 12, 797880. https://doi.org/10.3389/fimmu.2021.797880

11 Obesity and Cancer Risk: A Public Health Crisis (ajmc.com)

Chapter 17

1 Germans Baffled by Soccer Players Collapsing & Dropping Dead on the Field (independentsentinel.com)

2 Montgomery J, Ryan M, Engler R, et al. Myocarditis Following Immunization With mRNA COVID-19 Vaccines in Members of the US Military. JAMA Cardiol. 2021;6(10):1202–1206. doi:10.1001/jamacardio.2021.2833

3 Dionne A, Sperotto F, Chamberlain S, Baker AL, Powell AJ, Prakash A, Castellanos DA, Saleeb SF, de Ferranti SD, Newburger JW, Friedman KG. Association of Myocarditis With BNT162b2 Messenger RNA COVID-19 Vaccine in a Case Series of Children. JAMA Cardiol. 2021 Dec 1;6(12):1446-1450. doi: 10.1001/jamacardio.2021.3471. PMID: 34374740; PMCID: PMC8356143.

4 Jenna Schauer, Sujatha Buddhe, Jessica Colyer, Eyal Sagiv, Yuk Law, Sathish Mallenahalli Chikkabyrappa, Michael A. Portman, Myopericarditis After the Pfizer Messenger Ribonucleic Acid Coronavirus Disease Vaccine in Adolescents, The Journal of Pediatrics, Volume 238, 2021, Pages 317-320, ISSN 0022-3476, https://doi.org/10.1016/j.jpeds.2021.06.083.

5 Fazlollahi A, Zahmatyar M, Noori M, Nejadghaderi SA, Sullman MJM, Shekarriz-Foumani R, Kolahi AA, Singh K, Safiri S. Cardiac complications following mRNA COVID-19 vaccines: A systematic review of case reports and case series. Rev Med Virol. 2021 Dec 17:e2318. doi: 10.1002/rmv.2318. Epub ahead of print. PMID: 34921468.

6 Nygaard, Ulrikka PhD*; Holm, Mette PhD†; Bohnstedt, Cathrine PhD*; Chai, Qing PhD‡; Schmidt, Lisbeth Samsø PhD§; Hartling, Ulla Birgitte PhD¶; Petersen, Jens Jakob Herrche PhD||; Thaarup, Jesper PhD**; Bjerre, Jesper PhD†; Vejlstrup, Niels Grove PhD*; Juul, Klaus PhD*; Stensballe, Lone Graff PhD* Population-based Incidence of Myopericarditis After COVID-19 Vaccination in Danish Adolescents, The Pediatric Infectious Disease Journal: January 2022 - Volume 41 - Issue 1 - p e25-e28 doi: 10.1097/INF.0000000000003389

7 The Rio Times. Sept. 17, 2021. https://www.riotimesonline.com/brazil-news/modern-day-censorship/ncaa-golfer-has-severe-adverse-heart-condition-due-to-covid-vaccine-speaks-out-against-vaccine-mandates/. Retrieved August 14, 2022.

Chapter 18

1 Design and Analysis of Shedding Studies for Virus or Bacteria-Based Gene Therapy and Oncolytic Products - Guidance for Industry (fda.gov)

2 Richard Plasse, Robert Nee, Sanh Gao, Stephen Olson, Acute kidney injury with gross hematuria and IgA nephropathy after COVID-19 vaccination, Kidney International, Volume 100, Issue 4, 2021, Pages 944-945, ISSN 0085-2538, https://doi.org/10.1016/j.kint.2021.07.020.

3 Bleier BS, Ramanathan M, Lane AP. COVID-19 Vaccines May Not Prevent Nasal SARS-CoV-2 Infection and Asymptomatic Transmission. Otolaryngology–Head and Neck Surgery. 2021;164(2):305-307. doi:10.1177/0194599820982633

Chapter 19

1 Myofascial Pain and Dysfunction. The Trigger Point Manual. Volume 1: Upper Half of Body. Second edition, James J. Bergman, The Journal of the American Board of Family Practice. September 1999, 12 (5) 425; DOI: https://doi.org/10.3122/jabfm.12.5.425a

2 Suzuki, Y. J., & Gychka, S. G. (2021). SARS-CoV-2 Spike Protein Elicits Cell Signaling in Human Host Cells: Implications for Possible Consequences of COVID-19 Vaccines. Vaccines, 9(1), 36. https://doi.org/10.3390/vaccines9010036

3 http://dx.doi.org/10.1136/thoraxjnl-2021-217985

4 McLachlan, Scott & Osman, Magda & Dube, Kudakwashe & Chiketero, Patience & Choi, Yvonne & Fenton, Norman. (2021). Analysis of COVID-19 vaccine death reports from the Vaccine Adverse Events Reporting System (VAERS) Database Interim: Results and Analysis. 10.13140/RG.2.2.26987.26402.

Chapter 20

1 COVID: Children's extremely low risk confirmed by study - BBC News Clare Smith, David Odd, Rachel Harwood et al. Deaths in Children and Young People in England following SARS-CoV-2 infection during the first pandemic year: a national study using linked mandatory child death reporting data, 07 July 2021, PREPRINT (Version 1) available at Research Square [https://doi.org/10.21203/rs.3.rs-689684/v1]

2 Li X, Lai FTT, Chua GT, et al. Myocarditis Following COVID-19 BNT162b2 Vaccination Among Adolescents in Hong Kong. JAMA Pediatr. Published online February 25, 2022. doi:10.1001/jamapediatrics.2022.0101

3 Høeg, T. et al. (2021) "SARS-CoV-2 mRNA Vaccination-Associated Myocarditis in Children Ages 12-17: A Stratified National Database Analysis". *medRxiv*. Doi: 10.1101/2021.08.30.21262866.

4 Jenna Schauer, Sujatha Buddhe, Avanti Gulhane, Eyal Sagiv, Matthew Studer, Jessica Colyer, Sathish Mallenahalli Chikkabyrappa, Yuk Law, Michael A. Portman. Persistent Cardiac Magnetic Resonance Imaging Findings in a Cohort of Adolescents with Post-Coronavirus Disease 2019 mRNA Vaccine Myopericarditis, The Journal of Pediatrics, 2022, ISSN 0022-3476, https://doi.org/10.1016/j.jpeds.2022.03.032. Myocarditis in Children | Symptoms, Causes, Treatment & Prognosis (cincinnatichildrens.org)

5 Search Results from the VAERS Database (medalerts.org)

6 Risk of Myopericarditis following COVID-19 mRNA vaccination in a Large Integrated Health System: A Comparison of Completeness and Timeliness of Two Methods. Katie A Sharff, David M Dancoes, Jodi L Longueil, Eric S Johnson, Paul F Lewis. https://doi.org/10.1101/2021.12.21.21268209

7 https://www.wsj.com/articles/cdc-COVID-19-coronavirus-vaccine-side-effects-hospitalization-kids-11626706868, http://www.opensourcetruth.com/johns-hopkins-study-found-zero-COVID-deaths-among-healthy-kids/

8 Karrow NA, Shandilya UK, Pelech S, Wagter-Lesperance L, McLeod D, Bridle B, Mallard BA. Maternal COVID-19 Vaccination and Its Potential Impact on Fetal and Neonatal Development. *Vaccines*. 2021; 9(11):1351. https://doi.org/10.3390/vaccines9111351

9 https://abc7news.com/COVID-death-count-alameda-county-deaths-19-cases/10755419/, retrieved April 23, 2022

10 https://www.nbcboston.com/news/local/massachusetts-reports-significant-overcount-of-COVID-deaths/2665981/

11 https://www.euronews.com/my-europe/2020/08/13/coronavirus-uk-reduces-death-toll-by-5-000-as-it-revises-counting-strategy

12 Why are we vaccinating children against COVID-19? - ScienceDirect

13 https://www.folkhalsomyndigheten.se/the-public-health-agency-of-sweden/communicable-disease-control/COVID-19/vaccination-against-COVID-19/children-and-adolescents--information-about-vaccination-against-COVID-19/

14 https://www.sickkids.ca/contentassets/50c1bd3c95e74dcf9fa7c9f6fd707b-d7/interim-guidance_myocarditis-pericarditis-after-mrna-COVID-19-vaccination-in-children.pdf

15 Fact Sheet for Recipients - Pfizer-BioNTech COVID-19 Vaccine for 5 - 11 Years of Age (fda.gov)

Chapter 21

1 c19ivermectin.com, c19adoption.com

2 Obesity studies highlight severe COVID outcomes, even in young adults | CIDRAP (umn.edu)

3 Frank, R. C., Mendez, S. R., Stevenson, E. K., Guseh, J. S., Chung, M., & Silverman, M. G. (2020). Obesity and the Risk of Intubation or Death in Patients With Coronavirus Disease 2019. Critical care medicine, 48(11), e1097–e1101. https://doi.org/10.1097/CCM.0000000000004553

4 Djaharuddin, I., Munawwarah, S., Nurulita, A., Ilyas, M., Tabri, N. A., & Lihawa, N. (2021). Comorbidities and mortality in COVID-19 patients. Gaceta sanitaria, 35 Suppl 2, S530–S532. https://doi.org/10.1016/j.gaceta.2021.10.085

5 COVID-19-and-Obesity-The-2021-Atlas.pdf (worldobesityday.org)

6 Demeulemeester, F., de Punder, K., van Heijningen, M., & van Doesburg, F. (2021). Obesity as a Risk Factor for Severe COVID-19 and Complications: A Review. Cells, 10(4), 933. https://doi.org/10.3390/cells10040933

7 Mortality Analyses - Johns Hopkins Coronavirus Resource Center (jhu.edu)

8 Dessie, Z.G., Zewotir, T. Mortality-related risk factors of COVID-19: a systematic review and meta-analysis of 42 studies and 423,117 patients. BMC Infect Dis 21, 855 (2021). https://doi.org/10.1186/s12879-021-06536-3

9 Science, Public Health Policy, and The Law Volume 2:4-22 October 12, 2020 ETHICS IN SCIENCE AND TECHNOLOGY An Institute for Pure and Applied Knowledge (IPAK) Public Health Policy Initiative (PHPI) COVID-19 Data Collection, Comorbidity & Federal Law: A Historical Retrospective Henry Ealy * , † , Michael McEvoy ‡§, Daniel Chong , John Nowicki , Monica Sava, Sandeep Gupta k , David White **, James Jordan, Daniel Simon ††, Paul Anderson ‡‡

10 https://www.saveusnow.org.uk/COVID-vaccine-scientific-proof-lethal/

Resources and Support Sites

1 About the National Vaccine Injury Compensation Program | Official web site of the U.S. Health Resources & Services Administration (hrsa.gov)

2 McLachlan, Scott & Osman, Magda & Dube, Kudakwashe & Chiketero, Patience & Choi, Yvonne & Fenton, Norman. (2021). Analysis of COVID-19 vaccine death reports from the Vaccine Adverse Events Reporting System (VAERS) Database Interim: Results and Analysis. 10.13140/RG.2.2.26987.26402.

3 United States Department of Health and Human Services (DHHS), Public Health Service (PHS), Centers for Disease Control (CDC) / Food and Drug Administration (FDA), Vaccine Adverse Event Reporting System (VAERS) 1990 - 04/22/2022, CDC WONDER On-line Database. Accessed at http://wonder.cdc.gov/vaers.html on May 4, 2022 11:33:56 AM

4 United States Department of Health and Human Services (DHHS), Public Health Service (PHS), Centers for Disease Control (CDC) / Food and Drug Administration (FDA), Vaccine Adverse Event Reporting System (VAERS) 1990 - 04/22/2022, CDC WONDER On-line Database. Accessed at http://wonder.cdc.gov/vaers.html on May 4, 2022 11:42:37 AM

5 VAERS - Data (hhs.gov)

6 Abbasi J. COVID-19 and mRNA Vaccines-First Large Test for a New Approach. JAMA. 2020 Sep 22;324(12):1125-1127. doi: 10.1001/jama.2020.16866. PMID: 32880613.

7 https://www.thegms.co/medical-ethics/medethics-rw-22021403.pdf

About the Author

Deanna has been in the medical field for 35 years first as a United States Air Force Medic, then as a phlebotomist, EKG technician, Registered Nurse, Staff Educator/QI, and finally, an Adult-Geriatric Nurse Practitioner. She worked primarily in cardiac critical care intensive care, followed by home and hospice care, and more recently, primary care. She is grateful for a life of learning, teaching, and helping people find abundant healing in all aspects of life, based in Truth and exciting transformation of the mind, heart, body, relationships, and life. She enjoys sunshine, fresh air, and licorice. She deeply loves family, friends, and Jesus, Who, incredibly, loves us all.

Author Note

Thank you so much for reading Gasoline. I am so very grateful for you!

Please take a moment to leave a review to help other people know they are not alone, to know of the potential health concerns to watch for and hopefully be better able to find help toward healing. Reviews make a significant impact and adding yours can help reach other people. Again, many thanks to you!

Made in the USA
Middletown, DE
24 November 2022